DEDICATION

To my husband, Chris, who is always there for me,
through thick and thin. I love you so very much.

DISCLAIMER

The disclaimer is the "awkward conversation" we need to have at the outset to ensure we're on the same page.

This book contains my personal experiences, opinions, and advice. My statements are not intended to treat, diagnose, or cure any medical condition. I am not a doctor, lawyer, or licensed therapist. Neither my publisher nor I offer medical, legal, or psychological advice, and no contents of this book are to be construed as the advice, care, or treatment of a licensed professional, or as a substitute for such professional services.

This book contains my experiences with the HCG Diet. Diets and hormone therapies that are safe and appropriate for one person may be neither safe nor appropriate for another. Before undertaking any diet or hormone therapy on your own, consult with the appropriate professionals.

This book is offered "as-is", and my publisher and I disclaim all liability in connection with the use of it or its contents.

Use of this book implies your acceptance of this disclaimer.

BONUS MATERIAL

20 Tips to Rock Your HCG Diet

A Daily Weight Loss Affirmation

Dr. Simeons Book, Pounds and Inches

Author Videos

and

20 Essential Nutrition Habits for Permanent Weight Loss

Sign up at:

www.theHCGDietBook.com

ADELE FRIZZELL

CONTENTS

INTRODUCTION: CUTTING THROUGH THE HYPE

Welcome to The HCG Diet: Fact and Fiction.

I wrote this book because there is so much conflicting information regarding the controversial HCG Diet. Most of what is written about the HCG Diet is either fear mongering, or, the benefits are greatly exaggerated.

Perhaps you've seen the headlines:

- Lose 1 – 2 pounds a day!
- Lose fat evenly!
- Preserve muscle!
- Reset your metabolism!
- Improve thyroid function!
- Keep the weight off permanently!

…And so on.

I want to cut through the hype and expose the truth.

This is the book I wish I had purchased before starting my own HCG Diet journey: it would have saved me a lot of money, doubt, and struggle.

I speak from personal experience with the diet, having done four rounds, two of which were botched. I've tried the homeopathic drops, as well as prescription HCG pills and injections. I've had to terminate rounds early due to hunger and I've tried different protocols.

In total, I lost 28 pounds on the diet. It's the only diet that has ever worked for me, and I've been trying to lose weight for four years. I am, as they say, a "hard loser".

My persistence ultimately paid off, and I share the experience, along with my research, in an effort to answer every possible question about the diet: how it works, why it works, and what you can expect to happen to your body. I don't want you to struggle as much as I did to lose weight, keep it off, or choose a protocol and medication

> *Through trial and error, I found an approach that worked better for me than the original 500-claorie protocol. Although I don't go into detail about it in this book, my version doesn't require severe calorie restriction or eliminating whole food groups. It didn't require me to stop exercising. I was able to eat more, work out, and I still lost the same amount of weight. I wrote this book (and later became a certified health coach) to help people reach their physique goals in a way that is customized, scientific, and sustainable for them.*

Was the HCG Diet worth all the sacrifice? Absolutely, yes.

I finally achieved my goal of being in the 160s again after four years of trying to lose 25 - 30 pounds the slow and "sensible" way through 1) Following popular diets like Jenny Craig 2) Counting macros and calories, and 3) Healthier eating habits and "intuitive" eating. In those four years, I worked with a nutritionist, a coach, and a Registered Dietician but I could never lose more than ten pounds. I also couldn't keep the weight off for longer than a couple of weeks. My body seemed stuck at a certain weight and hunger always sabotaged my weight-loss efforts.

I truly believe that the hormone in the HCG Diet helps to balance hormones and suppress hunger, *if you are on the right dose*. For some folks, it completely suppresses their appetite. For others, it just turns the dial down enough to make dieting tolerable.

I am sure you have lots of questions about the diet, so let's get started. If you're brand new to the HCG Diet, then some of the terminology will be new to you. If that's the case, I recommend skipping to **Chapter 4: Important Terminology** and reading it first.

Let's get started!

Adele Frizzell

We fall for hype because what we really need is hope.

ADELE FRIZZELL

CHAPTER 1: THE CONTROVERSY

WHY ARE SO MANY PEOPLE AGAINST THE HCG DIET?

The HCG Diet is a controversial one. Although many people have experienced tremendous success on it, most experts, including the FDA, believe it is ineffective for weight loss and carries considerable health risks.

And yet, tens of thousands of people, including myself, have lost weight safely and (relatively) easily on the HCG Diet.

As a result, we seem to have an irreconcilable and incredible difference of opinion.

WHAT'S YOUR OPINION OF THE HCG DIET?

People seem to be divided into four camps or opinions when it comes to the HCG diet.

Camp One: Those with overwhelmingly positive opinions of the HCG Diet based on direct personal experience. This includes:

1. Doctors who have successfully helped hundreds or even thousands of patients lose weight.

2. Dieters who have tried everything else only to finally lose weight on the HCG Diet.

Camp Two: Those with overwhelmingly negative opinions of the HCG Diet based on direct personal experience. This includes:

1. Unsuccessful dieters who became ravenous and couldn't follow the diet. They feel understandably let-down and frustrated. They may have been unaware that finding the correct dosage of HCG – neither too much nor too little – makes all the difference as far as hunger is concerned. This was my situation; it took time to figure out the correct medication and dosage.

2. Unsuccessful dieters who suffered adverse side effects such as weakness, leg cramping, insomnia, and electrolyte imbalances. They may have been unaware that certain vitamins could have helped, and a higher-calorie protocol may have reduced or eradicated these side effects. *

*I discuss a more detailed list of potential side effects in Chapter 2.

Camp Three: The opinionated masses with no personal experience. This includes:

1. People who haven't tried the HCG Diet but heard it was dangerous, and thus formed a baseless opinion about it with no research or experience.

2. People who have enough knowledge of nutrition to know that rapid weight-loss diets are rarely successful and

consuming less than 1200 calories a day is ill-advised.

These two groups of people often can't understand why someone wouldn't just change their eating habits and try to lose weight the "safe" way.

I'll confess: until I tried the HCG Diet myself, I fell in Camp 3.

Camp Four: The scientists and experts. This includes:

1. Nutritionists.

2. The FDA.

While I have the utmost respect for nutritionists and scientists, I do believe their personal reservations and conclusions are entirely due to a lack of quality-controlled studies on the hormone.

Let me explain.

In 1995, a meta-analysis (a statistical analysis which crunches the data on many separate but related studies) analyzed 24 trials of the HCG Diet over a period of decades. They determined that 16 of the studies were uncontrolled and 8 were controlled. The researchers also determined that only 12 of the studies were of sufficient statistical quality to be usable. Of those 12 that made the cut, only one of those studies indicated that the HCG Diet was useful. From the meta-analysis, it was concluded that the HCG Diet was not effective. *

*Source: *https://www.ncbi.nlm.nih.gov/pmc/articles/PMC1365103*

Fair enough.

But it is important to note that all the studies were based on the original 500-calorie Simeons Protocol. Presumably, they would have used injections of 125 IU. This is a crucial point because a lot of people struggle with hunger until they find the right dose, which could be anywhere between 125 and 250 IU. Also, many people nowadays are choosing to do higher-calorie protocols (anywhere from 650 – 1200 calories a day). Although fewer than 1000 calories a day is still considered a "starvation diet", more calories do provide more nutrients to the body and help reduce the risk of electrolyte imbalances.

THE FDA'S POSITION ON THE HCG DIET

Currently, the FDA's stance on the HCG Diet is that:

> *"HCG has not been demonstrated to be effective adjunctive therapy in the treatment of obesity. There is no substantial evidence beyond that resulting from caloric restriction, that it causes a more attractive or 'normal' distribution of fat, or that it decreases the hunger and discomfort associated with calorie-restricted diets."*

It's also worth noting that the HCG Diet isn't exactly *banned* but nor is it *approved*. What is illegal is the use of HCG Diet *products* sold in the form of oral drops, pellets, and sprays.

> *The FDA considers new drugs to be unsafe until they are proven safe through clinical trials, typically funded by pharmaceutical companies. And this is the problem in a nutshell…*

For a drug to be "approved" by the U.S. Food and Drug Administration (FDA), it must be deemed safe and effective through rigorous trials. The FDA must also decide if the benefits of the approved item outweigh the potential risks for the item's planned use.

Since the FDA doesn't conduct its own trials, it relies on the research provided by the drug companies. It then uses its own experts (statisticians, biologists, chemists, and physicians) to analyze the data presented from the manufacturer. Based on this analysis, the FDA decides whether to approve a drug.

Can you see the problem? There is no drug company conducting controlled studies in live human subjects on the use of HCG as a weight-loss aid. Due to a lack of rigorous scientific research (as mentioned at the beginning of this chapter, the studies we do have are mostly small and poorly conducted), the FDA cannot approve HCG for use as a weight-loss aid.

However, the FDA does permit HCG as a prescription medication to treat fertility issues. From the FDA website:

> *HCG is FDA-approved for the treatment of select cases of female infertility and hormone*

treatment in men. FDA-approved HCG products are only available in injection-form and require a prescription from a licensed medical professional.

Officially, HCG is not "approved" for over-the-counter use as a weight-loss product and this includes homeopathic drops. At the time of this writing, the FDA is actively taking legal action against companies that sell homeopathic drops online.

As for prescription HCG, "the FDA is aware that healthcare professionals sometimes prescribe prescription injectable HCG for unapproved uses such as weight loss." * This is deemed off-label use and it appears to be a grey area for the FDA.

*Source:
https://www.fda.gov/Drugs/ResourcesForYou/Consumers/BuyingUsing MedicineSafely/MedicationHealthFraud/ucm281834.htm

The FDA does state on its website that consuming a 500-calorie diet to lose weight is potentially dangerous. They are concerned that consumers may not get enough vitamins, minerals, and protein, and the risks that can occur as a result. Chiefly, an increased risk for "gallstone formation, an imbalance of the electrolytes that keep the body's muscles and nerves functioning properly, and an irregular heartbeat." * Regardless, the FDA's caution and my own research and knowledge of nutrition explains, in part, why I prefer a higher-calorie, higher-protein approach.

*Source:
https://www.fda.gov/ForConsumers/ConsumerUpdates/ucm281333.htm

MY OWN CONCLUSIONS

I am not a doctor, nutritionist, or scientist. The FAQs in the next chapter are based on my own personal experience (on which I rely most heavily), and information gathered from various sources: my personal DXA scans, lab results, patient forums, PubMed* articles, books, blogs, and conversations with a nutritionist, and a doctor who prescribes HCG for weight loss.

DXA Scan: The most accurate method for determining a person's total body composition (muscle, bone, and body fat percentage) is a DXA scan. DXA stands for Dual Energy X-ray Absorptiometry. Other popular methods such as skinfold testing and bio-impedance devices are much less accurate at determining a person's body fat.

PubMed: PubMed comprises more than 27 million citations for biomedical literature. It is the go-to resource for doctors and health professionals.

Based on this research, I _agree_ with the FDA's stance in regard to the following:

1. The diet does not cause a "more attractive or 'normal' distribution of fat". This is akin to spot reducing, which has been debunked.

The diet simply means you will draw from fat stores as an energy source when calories are insufficient. You will reduce more in some areas and less in others based on your genetics. I experienced this personally as I appeared to lose more fat from my legs and arms and face. This uneven distribution of fat loss was verified when I had some DXA scans done of my body. The printouts revealed that I lost more fat in my legs than my belly region, even though my legs were leaner, and I had more fat to lose in my belly (I have an apple shape). If my bodyfat was supposed to become more "normal" or "attractive" as per the marketing hype, I should have lost a greater percentage of fat tissue around my abdomen.

However, I *disagree* with the FDA's stance as far as hunger is concerned:

1. "HCG has not been demonstrated to be effective adjunctive therapy in the treatment of obesity."

I believe the diet does help people lose weight, and it can be an effective treatment for obesity, when used in conjunction with lifestyle and behavior modifications to maintain a weight loss.

2. The FDA states that there is no substantial evidence that HCG will decrease "the hunger and discomfort associated with calorie-restricted diets".

If that were the case, why has hunger sabotaged every

other diet I've tried in the last four years but not this one?

I believe the HCG hormone does impact hunger (and so do thousands of other people) but I can only speculate as to why. One very plausible theory is that the HCG hormone acts on leptin* to reduce hunger while dieting. Another is that it balances hormones. Interestingly, my thyroid labs showed an improvement in function while taking HCG, and I eventually had to lower my thyroid dose because I started to feel hyper. This is quite extraordinary as one of the negative consequences of prolonged dieting and/or rapid weight loss is the exact opposite effect: a *decrease* in thyroid function over time. It is noteworthy that after the diet ended, and six months had passed, I started to feel some hypothyroid symptoms return. I increased my thyroid dose again but never went back to previous levels.

*Source: *Weight-Loss Apocalypse: Emotional Eating Rehab Through the HCG Protocol by Robin Phipps Woodall*

I believe more research is needed to fully appreciate the impact of the hormone, and the diet itself. I would love to see some research done on higher-calorie protocols, and more studies which take into account the efficacy of different dosages and forms of HCG (homeopathic drops versus injection versus oral pellets.) Surely, there are some undergraduates out there looking for a thesis topic? (Hint hint.)

Until more studies are done, I believe personal experience, and the sum testimony of patients and physicians is the best evidence available at this time. This is because it is based on the direct experience of thousands of patients versus small trials.

It can take one dedicated scientist to turn the tide of public opinion. For example, not too long ago, it was commonly believed that stress causes ulcers. It is now known that it is caused by a bacterium. But until Dr. Barry Marshall ingested the bacteria in 1985 to prove his point, no one would believe him, not even other scientists, who were very dismissive when he and his partner, Robin Warren began their research. Dr. Marshall's sacrifice and dedication to this discovery helped his team win the Nobel Peace Prize in 2005 and put an end to ulcers in Australia.

In any case, I hope this book sparks more intelligent conversation and research into the HCG Diet. Whether or not the hormone has the potential to "cure" obesity requires more study.

What else are we convinced we know that we don't?

Only humility, curiosity, and a willingness to experiment with an open mind will allow us to advance our knowledge.

CHAPTER 2: HCG DIET FAQ

The goal of this chapter is to answer the more common questions when it comes to the HCG Diet.

Please note that this information may become outdated or inaccurate as knowledge of nutrition and the HCG hormone evolves. If you have a question I haven't answered below, please email me at CoachingWithAdele@gmail.com. I may update future editions of this book with your questions.

WHAT IS THE HCG DIET?

Q: What is the HCG Diet?

The HCG Diet is a rapid weight-loss diet. In a nutshell, patients take HCG* hormone medication every day for approximately three weeks (a short round) or six weeks (a long round) while normally consuming 500 - 1000 calories a day and eating from a list of restricted foods. That list of restricted foods and the number of calories you can eat depends on which version of the HCG Diet you wish to follow. There are several versions of the diet out there (see Terminology section) but the original diet was created by Dr. Simeons more than 70 years ago.

*HCG = *human chorionic gonadotropin hormone.*

The Original Simeons Protocol

Dr. Simeons pioneered the original HCG Diet in the 1950s after successfully treating thousands of obese patients at his in-patient clinic in Rome, Italy. Daily injections of HCG (125 IU) were given and dieters were restricted to less than 500 calories a day. They were only allowed to eat from a small list of permitted foods and no fats were permitted during the diet phase.

Thousands of people still follow the original protocol as outlined in Dr. Simeons book, *Pounds and Inches*. If you sign up for my mailing list, I will send you a free copy. Visit www.TheHCGDietBook.com.

How is the HCG Diet different from other crash diets?

Q: How is the HCG diet different from other crash diets?

After all, anyone restricting their daily intake to 25 - 50% of the recommended daily allowance WILL lose weight. There's nothing especially magical about that, right? That's what the critics say, and they're right. Provided you can stay on it, if you follow a 500 - 1000 calorie diet you will lose a lot of weight – rapidly. But while the critics are focused on the "Diet" part of the HCG Diet, they are missing the most crucial component: the "HCG".

On the HCG Diet, human chorionic gonadotropin hormone is taken in combination with a specific diet to lose weight rapidly. It is believed that the HCG hormone acts on leptin* to reduce hunger while dieting.

*Source: *Weight-Loss Apocalypse: Emotional Eating Rehab Through the HCG Protocol by Robin Phipps Woodall*

Without **real HCG**, it would be virtually impossible to live on 500 - 1000 calories a day and function at a high level. You would feel incredibly lethargic, have brain fog, and feel hungry all the time. Eventually the wheels would come off and you'd find yourself binging (as I did, on the homeopathic drops). A person can only fight their biology for so long.

In fact, the hormone is why some people prefer to call the HCG Diet a "Hormone protocol" or "HCG Medication Therapy".

> *It took a few hundred cases to establish beyond reasonable doubt that the mechanism operates in exactly the same way and seemingly without exception in every case of obesity…. most patients complained that the two meals of 250 calories each were more than they could manage, as they continually had a feeling of just having had a large meal.*
>
> - Dr. Simeons, *Pounds and Inches*

WHAT IS HCG?

Q: What is HCG?

Human chorionic gonadotropin hormone (HCG) is a hormone that is produced by the human placenta during pregnancy. It helps pregnant women to nurture the growing fetus even when calories are absent. The hormone prioritizes nutrients to help the baby grow, even if the mother is starving, by drawing from her fat stores when insufficient calories are present.

> *Ideal nutritional conditions for the fetus can only be achieved when the mother's blood is continually saturated with food, regardless of whether she eats or not, as otherwise a period of starvation might hamper the steady growth of the embryo. It seems that HCG brings about this continual saturation of the blood, which is the reason why obese patients under treatment with HCG never feel hungry in spite of their drastically reduced food intake.*
>
> - Dr. Simeons, *Pounds and Inches*

WHAT IS LEPTIN AND HOW DOES IT WORK?

Q: What is leptin and how does it work?

There are no foods that contain leptin. Leptin is a protein hormone that's made in the fat cells. It circulates in the bloodstream and goes to the brain. It plays a crucial role in appetite and weight control as well as energy regulation and long-term fat storage.

Discovered in 1994, leptin is often referred to as the fat hormone, obesity hormone and/or starvation hormone.

WHAT IS LEPTIN RESISTANCE?

Q: What is leptin resistance?

Since leptin is made in the fat cells, you would think overweight and obese people have adequate levels of this hormone (low levels trigger hunger). However, the term "leptin resistant" was coined in obese subjects who have enough (or more than enough) leptin freely circulating in their bloodstream – their body just can't utilize it.

There are two hypotheses behind leptin resistance. The first is that leptin in the blood is not crossing the blood-brain barrier to bind to receptors in the area of the brain that controls appetite. The other theory is that the receptors themselves aren't functioning properly.

In both scenarios, we have a communication breakdown.

If the brain senses low leptin levels, regardless of cause (either through dieting or through leptin resistance), then intense food cravings and constant hunger will result. It's also worth noting that low leptin levels also encourage fat storage.

WHO IS AT RISK FOR LEPTIN RESISTANCE?

Q: Who is at risk for leptin resistance?

The cause of leptin resistance is inconclusive, though genetics and years of overeating may play a role. The more overweight or obese you are, the more at risk you are of developing leptin resistance. Leptin resistance goes hand in hand with insulin resistance, which is a driving factor leading to diabetes.

The good news? Since leptin is created and stored in fatty tissue, losing excess fat may restore some of the body's sensitivity to the hormone and reverse or reduce the effects of insulin resistance. Studies have also shown that exercise can restore leptin sensitivity. *

*Source:
http://journals.plos.org/plosbiology/article?id=10.1371%2Fjournal.pbio.1000465#s3

Better regulation and utilization of leptin means a reduction in hunger and cravings, and the ability to maintain a healthier body weight with greater ease.

However, improved leptin regulation doesn't address the deeper issues of emotional eating, constant overeating in the absence of hunger, and poor eating habits. The consequences of these behaviors, if left unchecked, will continue to sabotage all weight loss efforts.

This is what makes fat loss so difficult: there are genetic, environmental, behavioral, and psychological contributors that need to be addressed if the goal is to maintain a healthy weight for life.

HOW MUCH WEIGHT CAN I EXPECT TO LOSE?

Q: How much weight can I expect to lose on the HCG Diet?

You can expect to lose anywhere from 5 - 15 pounds in your first week and then 2 - 5 pounds every week thereafter.

Women typically lose 15 - 30 pounds in a six-week round, and men lose more: 20 - 40 pounds is not unusual. * I personally lost 21 pounds in six weeks on roughly 1000 calories a day using my own higher-calorie, higher-protein protocol. This is average for a female (an average of half pound a day). The more fat you have to lose, the better your results will be.

Males typically lose more than females due to a higher basal metabolic rate (BMR). Patients who take thyroid medication typically lose a little less than average.

CAN I DO THE HCG DIET IF I ONLY HAVE TO LOSE 5 – 10 POUNDS?

Q: Can I do the HCG Diet if I only have to lose 5 – 10 pounds?

Although Dr. Simeons would treat patients with as little as five pounds to lose, the HCG Diet was created for obese patients and is best suited for individuals with more than ten pounds to lose. Personally, I suggest some behavioral changes and healthier eating habits if you are within striking distance of your ideal weight.

Whether you only have a few pounds to lose, or you have lost the weight and wish to maintain your new body weight for life, I recommend Georgie Fear's book, *Lean Habits for Lifelong Weight Loss: Mastering Four Core Eating Behaviors to Stay Slim Forever.* It's a terrific book from a well-respected Registered Dietician.

Is the HCG Diet expensive?

Q: Is the HCG Diet expensive?

The medication is the costliest part of the HCG Diet, but your reduced food costs will offset this. You will save a lot of money by not eating out, going to coffee shops, or buying a lot of groceries while you're on the diet.

If you order your HCG product online, it should be less than $300 a month for a prescription, and less than $400 for two months. If you visit a doctor's clinic, your costs could easily exceed $1000 a month for the bloodwork, medication, and visits.

Where do I buy HCG?

Q: Where Do I Buy HCG?

You can purchase prescription HCG online or through a medical weight-loss center. I provide the names of a couple places from which I purchased prescription HCG, but I am in no way affiliated with them at the time of this publication. I only mention the names of these suppliers to provide you with some options if you're shopping online.

Regardless of which vendor you choose to order your product from, it's extremely important to purchase only real HCG from a company that uses an FDA certified compounding pharmacy. You must buy the purest HCG you can if you want to lose weight rapidly and keep hunger at bay while consuming a meagre number of calories. Real HCG can mean the difference between success and failure, and I have experienced both first-hand. (More on this in a moment.)

I've personally purchased and used HCG in the following forms:

- Injections
- Oral Drops
- Oral Pellets

I had injections done at a medical weight-loss clinic four years ago, and I lost 17 pounds in a month. (I slowly regained all the weight over a one-year period because I didn't have a plan for when the diet was over and resorted to old eating habits.)

I purchased homeopathic drops online through a Canadian supplier and lost a net 7 pounds in three weeks. I had to terminate that round early due to uncontrollable hunger.

I purchased oral pellets and lost an additional 21 pounds in six weeks. The oral pellets were purchased from two U.S. companies: NuImageMedical.com and DietDoc.com.

My Experience with NuImageMedical.com and DietDoc.com

Both NuImageMedical.com and DietDoc.com provide telemedicine and everything can be conveniently arranged via their website and over the phone. After speaking with a salesperson and completing a brief questionnaire online, I had a quick phone consultation with a nurse at NuImageMedical.com the next day, and a doctor at DietDoc.com that same day. Based on the information given, a prescription was approved. Note that I only paid for my medication, not the consultation, as consultations are free.

At the time of this writing, NuImageMedical.com provides customers with either a 23-day or 46-day prescription while DietDoc.com provides people with a 30-day or 60-day prescription. Prices vary, and the companies also follow different dietary protocols. NuImageMedical.com adheres to the original 500-calorie Simeons Protocol with a three or six-week round, while DietDoc.com prescribes a higher-calorie, higher-protein customized ketogenic approach and 30 or 60-day rounds. DietDoc.com also offers a nutritionist's help free of charge.

HCG DietDoc.com and NuImageMedical.com both use a

US based, FDA inspected compounding pharmacy for their prescriptions and this is essential to ensure the safety and purity of your medication.

Unfortunately, some products that are sold online and overseas contain only trace amounts of HCG and some contain none. There is no way to ensure the efficacy of a product if it doesn't come from a legitimate and approved pharmacy.

Pros and Cons of Injections, Drops, and Pellets

A brief description of the advantages and disadvantages of doing injections, drops, and pellets is listed below.

Injections

You can choose to inject yourself (normally once a day in the abdomen, alternating left and right sides a couple inches away from the belly button) or have a doctor or nurse do it for you at a clinic. Since it's inconvenient to have to visit a doctor's office every day, most people purchase their supplies online and opt to mix them and inject themselves at home. The needle is very tiny so the injection itself is pain-free. The medication also needs to be kept refrigerated after mixing, because it will lose potency if stored at room temperature longer than six hours. Injections always bring a risk of contamination so be sure to use alcohol swabs and bacteriostatic water.

A typical kit will include:

- A vial of pharmaceutical HCG (human chorionic gonadotropin) in powdered form
- Bacteriostatic water
- Mixing syringe
- Subcutaneous syringes
- Alcohol prep pads
- An instruction brochure

When I did the injections, I would visit my doctor once every two weeks. At that time, she would weigh me, answer any questions I had, and provide me with a 2-week supply of pre-loaded syringes. I would transport the syringes with ice packs to my fridge. During my check-ups, I was also given a B-12 shot in my upper right buttock, to help with flagging energy. It was an intramuscular shot, and it bruised and hurt a bit. The HCG injections used a much smaller needle and they were painless. I would inject myself at home.

Dr. Simeons only prescribed injections of 125 IU and some doctors still follow the original protocol religiously. This is unfortunate, as 125 IU could be too low for some people. Europeans were shorter and smaller (in general) in the 1950s, and probably needed less medication then. I see no reason for modern doctors to stick to this dosage and not adjust it for the individual's size or needs: 125-200 IU is usually sufficient for most individuals.

Advantages of Injections: You can be very precise and

personalized with the dosage and easily adjust it as needed. You can also consume food with your medication.

Disadvantages of Injections: Hassle of mixing and storing product in the fridge, risk of contamination, and risk of infection from injection site. The product quickly loses potency and should (ideally) be used up within two weeks of mixing. However, I spoke with a pharmacist who told me it is possible to store the mixed product for up to 30 days and still have satisfactory results.

You also need to find a safe way to dispose of your syringes. They shouldn't just be disposed of in the garbage, but at pharmacies, fire stations, or hospitals that take back syringes and biohazards.

If you decide to use a bricks-and-mortar clinic, you will be required to make doctor appointments which may require time off work.

Oral Drops

Drops are usually placed under the tongue and held for at least 30 seconds to get fully absorbed. People usually take 10 - 15 drops at a time, 3 - 4x a day. Some solutions may be mixed with other ingredients to increase energy or suppress appetite.

Advantages of Drops: Easy to administer and adjust dosage up or down as needed. No need to refrigerate: simply store in a cool, dark place away from sunlight or the microwave.

Disadvantages of Drops: Easy to take too much or too little, inconvenience of having to consume 3 - 4x a day, easy to forget to take the drops at specific times. The product will expire within one month once the bottle is opened so you can't save unused amounts for future rounds.

Oral Pellets

Oral pellets are referred to as troches when the pills are circular lozenges, individually separated in a package. Both the pellets and troches are designed to dissolve in your mouth in a matter of seconds. This allows the drug to get into your bloodstream quickly through the capillaries in your tongue and cheek.

Swallowing the medication before it is fully dissolved will reduce its effectiveness. This is because the digestion process reduces absorption.

Oral pellets/troches do not need to be refrigerated; however, they should not be exposed to heat above 85 degrees Fahrenheit/30 degrees Celsius. They normally have a 12-month shelf-life when stored at room temperature. However, always be sure to check the expiry date of your product.

Oral HCG medication typically contains 500 IU of HCG and should be compounded at an FDA-approved pharmacy through a doctor's prescription. The reason they contain so much HCG is that while some of the hormone enters the bloodstream through the capillaries, a portion of it is inevitably swallowed in the saliva, which reduces its effectiveness. Injections, on the other hand, go straight into the bloodstream.

I found the oral tablets to be the most convenient way to take the hormone. However, once I lost 25 pounds, the 500 IU dose became too high for me. I got all the classic pregnancy symptoms: my breasts swelled, and hunger and cravings became an issue. I tried to reduce my dosage by cutting the pellets, but this was too imprecise.

Advantages of Pellets: Long shelf-life, easy to take, great for travelers, only need to take once a day. No need to refrigerate. You can store any unused product for later use on another round (my tablets from DietDoc.com were labelled with an expiry date that was 14 months away). The pills don't need to be swallowed: they dissolve under the tongue in seconds.

Disadvantages of Pellets: According to a pharmacist I spoke to, you should take the oral pellets/troches an hour before eating anything, or two hours after your last meal. This is because the medication is most effective on an empty stomach and even if you dissolve the pill completely in your mouth, some of it will be invariably swallowed through saliva.

Perhaps the biggest disadvantage is that each pill has a set amount of HCG (normally 500 IU) so you can't adjust the dose up or down as needed. You could use a pill cutter, but that is imprecise. What if your sweet spot for dosing is 400 IU? And if your pills are teeny-tiny, as mine were from NuImageMedical.com, it won't be possible to cut them in half or quarters because they are the size of peppercorns and disintegrate easily.

Note: Always consult with your physician before adjusting your dosage.

If you are comfortable with injections but concerned about traveling with them and keeping them refrigerated, you could order a combination of injections and pills. This way, you get the benefit of precision through the injections, but you can use the pills for when you travel.

WHAT WORKS BETTER? INJECTIONS, DROPS, OR PELLETS?

My Personal Experience on Prescription HCG

I've purchased prescription HCG, in compounded pill form from two different US-based pharmacies. My first order came from NuImageMedical.com and my second order came from DietDoc.com. I found both prescriptions to be very effective. I did three weeks of sublingual pellets with NuImageMedical.com and three weeks of sublingual troches with DietDoc.com.

Four years ago, I did HCG injections through a bricks-and-mortar weight-loss clinic and lost 17 pounds (net) in a month. I followed the original Simeons Protocol and was 100% compliant. My only "cheat" was a Diet Pepsi every day.

While I lost similar amounts of weight on the oral pellets, I believe the injections are superior because you can be very precise with the dosage. As I mentioned, once I lost 25 pounds, the oral pellets became too high a dose for me.

It is worth noting that HCG injections are the only form of human chorionic gonadotropin hormone medication that is approved by the FDA.

Personal Experience on Homeopathic Drops

I had an open mind when I tried the drops. I liked that they were relatively inexpensive, the company seemed trustworthy, and many people had reportedly lost weight on them.

However, the wheels started coming off after the first week and I had to terminate my round early due to extreme hunger. It was a big waste of time and money and effort, not to mention a huge disappointment. This is why I cannot recommend drops, or a particular supplier when it comes to buying drops. While many people have successfully lost weight using the drops, my own experience, along with the negative experiences of friends and the FDA's stance on them means I cannot recommend them.

It's worth noting that although my supplier claimed the drops had real HCG, and their product was manufactured in an FDA approved lab, my hunger only went away once I switched to prescription HCG pellets.

HOW DO YOU KNOW WHAT IS REAL HCG AND WHAT IS FAKE?

Q: How do you know what is real HCG and what is fake?

There are some tip-offs as to whether a product contains real HCG or not:

1. If a doctor's prescription isn't required, it's not real HCG (at least in the U.S. and Canada). The real stuff should come from an FDA-approved pharmacy, and these pharmacies require a doctor's prescription. Like any prescription, the packaging should have your name and your doctor's name on it.

2. If the label or manufacturer says, "proprietary HCG", you should also treat it as a red flag. It is basically a blend of ingredients, some of which may help suppress the appetite, but it won't be as effective as real HCG.

3. The fake stuff is cheap. For example, you can buy "HCG Drops" at Walmart for $20. These imposters claim to do all the things real HCG does, but when you look closely at the ingredients, they usually say, "Proprietary Blend" or "HCG" in all caps.

4. "Human chorionic gonadotropin hormone" is not even a listed ingredient. However, my own homeopathic drops listed human chorionic gonadotropin as an ingredient, so consider point 1 in this list before anything else. I can only presume that if the drops did contain real HCG, then the amounts were insufficient. It's also worth mentioning that the drops did not give a positive result on a pregnancy test. More on this later.

5. The real stuff is expensive by comparison. A 30-day

supply is around $250 versus $20 for the drops.

HOMEOPATHIC HCG

Homeopathic HCG work on a different principle than pharmacy-grade HCG. Some people prefer it because they think it's more natural and they don't trust western medicine. They also don't like the thought of putting a hormone in their body. However, much of the homeopathic HCG that is sold online contains proprietary ingredients that may include trace amounts of HCG, lipotropic herbs, amino acids, metabolic boosters, and even appetite suppressants which aren't "natural" either. The drop market is essentially a free-for-all that attracts predatory individuals looking to benefit from a 30-billion-dollar supplement industry. It should also be noted that large studies have found homeopathy to be no more effective than a placebo.

From the FDA website:

> The Food and Drug Administration (FDA) is advising consumers to steer clear of these "homeopathic" human chorionic gonadotropin (HCG) weight-loss products. They are sold in the form of oral drops, pellets and sprays and can be found online and in some retail stores.
>
> FDA and the Federal Trade Commission (FTC) have issued seven letters to companies warning them that they are selling illegal

homeopathic HCG weight-loss drugs that have not been approved by FDA, and that make unsupported claims.

A reference document called the Homeopathic Pharmacopoeia of the United States lists active ingredients that may be legally included in homeopathic drug products.

HCG is not on this list and cannot be sold as a homeopathic medication for any purpose.

Source:
https://www.fda.gov/ForConsumers/ConsumerUpdates/ucm281333.htm

Potions Will Vary

Homeopathic HCG may or may not contain trace amounts of HCG, whereas fake HCG may contain nothing more than tap water or a proprietary blend of ingredients that has no HCG at all. As you can see, the lines are quite blurry.

That said, many people have experienced weight loss on homeopathic drops. Whether this is due to a placebo effect, or simply a low hunger drive and a lot of will power, we simply can't say. Some people really believe in homeopathy; I have the humility to accept that it may work, but I am skeptical that it is as effective as prescription HCG. It is also worth mentioning that customers who use the drops may miss out on the metabolic and hormonal benefits of the HCG hormone. (More on that later.)

Homeopathic drops seem to work best for those individuals who only have a little weight to lose.

MEDICAL CONSIDERATIONS

Q: Can anyone do this diet?

FDA warnings aside, both men and women can take human chorionic gonadotropin hormone, under a doctor's supervision. From the original book, *Pounds and Inches* by Dr. Simeons:

> *It cannot he sufficiently emphasized that HCG is not sex-hormone...HCG regulates menstruation and facilitates conception, but it never virilizes a woman or feminizes a man. It neither makes men grow breasts nor does it interfere with their virility, though where this was deficient it may improve it. It never makes women grow a beard or develop a gruff voice.*

> - Dr. Simeons, *Pounds and Inches*

However, the HCG Diet is not recommended for anyone under the age of 18, pregnant or breast-feeding women. If you are currently taking hormone therapy, or have an eating disorder such as anorexia, bulimia, or significant health problems such as cancer, epilepsy, heart disease, kidney disease, liver disease, or uncontrolled diabetes, then you should consult with your doctor or health care provider before starting the program.

If you haven't had a physical examination within the last year, I recommend getting one before starting the diet.

While human chorionic gonadotropin hormone has not been proven to cause cancer, it may aggravate existing cancer cells, fibroids, and tumors.

Also, if you are taking any type of medication, you may need to modify your prescription and/or dosage.

I'M A HARD LOSER, WILL THIS DIET STILL WORK FOR ME?

Q: I'm a hard loser, will this diet still work for me?

The HCG Diet has worked very well for hard losers (like me), menopausal women (like myself), those with thyroid issues (like myself), and those with PCOS and Type II diabetes (under a doctor's supervision).

WILL MY CHOLESTEROL IMPROVE?

Q: Will my cholesterol improve?

According to Lara Plagman, author of the book, *HCG Diet Options: Choosing Your Own Protocol,* people could see a "10%

decrease in LDL cholesterol and a 20 to 30% decrease in triglycerides." My own cholesterol improved, and my doctor was very pleased. However, this lowering of cholesterol, LDL, and triglycerides appears typical of diets that are low in saturated fats. *

*In this study, all 5 diets that were low in saturated fats lowered total cholesterol, LDL, and triglycerides.

Source:
https://www.ncbi.nlm.nih.gov/pubmed/30053283?dopt=Abstract

WILL I DAMAGE MY METABOLISM?

Q: Will the HCG Diet damage my metabolism?

The short answer is no, if you don't diet too long.

The long answer is that it is very difficult to permanently damage your metabolism on any diet, and this concept is really overhyped.

A study published in the journal, Metabolism, looked at over 400 overweight or obese women between 50 and 75 years of age with a history of yo-yo dieting. They concluded that moderate or severe weight cycling does not seem to impact the body's ability to lose weight, nor does it impact levels of hunger hormones or insulin sensitivity. *

*Source:
https://www.medicinenet.com/script/main/art.asp?articlekey=161490

What happens during a diet is that the body normally undergoes certain physiological and hormonal adaptions in response to fat loss. The changes include elevated cortisol and ghrelin (the hunger hormone), decreased energy, testosterone, thyroid, insulin, and leptin (the satiety hormone, or "fat hormone"). In essence, this is the body "pushing back" on weight loss and driving people to eat more and move less in an attempt to regain the weight being lost.

The longer people stay in a caloric deficit, the more these metabolic adaptations will hamper their weight-loss efforts. However, these adaptations are normal, and do not mean someone's metabolism is broken or slow just because losing weight is so difficult and the body keeps wanting to push back. As they say, "The struggle is real". Once a diet ends and enough calories are eaten to maintain a healthy bodyweight, normal metabolic functions resumes.

> *It should be noted that a very low-calorie diet has the potential to cause more severe adaptations than one that reduces calories only slightly, which is why I am more comfortable with higher-calorie, higher-protein versions of the HCG Diet.*

That said, our bodies are amazingly resilient. As hunter

gatherers, we were designed to go through periods of feast and famine. In fact, our modern habit of consuming three meals a day plus snacks and liquid calories is a big reason many of us are so overweight: we have never, in history, had access to so many calories and demanded so little of ourselves, physically.

Our bodies are amazingly resilient, and if you go into this diet in a relatively healthy state and limit yourself to a round no longer than 60 days, you should be fine. However, there are no guarantees in life, which is why you should never do this diet without a doctor's supervision, especially if you wish to do a longer round, or multiple rounds.

So where does this idea of "damaging" your metabolism and regaining all the weight again come from?

Well, you're more at risk of "damaging" your metabolism if, once the HCG Diet is over, you:

1. Continue to undereat possibly out of fear of regaining all the weight you lost.

2. Go through multiple rounds of the HCG Diet as way to counteract the problems of overeating – basically, going through extreme cycles of binging and undereating.

You will also likely regain the weight if you:

3. Neglect to adjust your new caloric intake to match your new bodyweight and activity level.

Keep in mind that a person who weighs 200 pounds often has a higher resting metabolic rate and can normally eat more calories than a smaller person. Therefore, if you could eat 2500 calories in the past and not gain weight, you may only be able to eat 2000 at your new bodyweight. This doesn't mean you damaged your metabolism, only that you are a smaller person now, and your caloric needs have decreased. If you want to eat 2500 calories again without gaining fat, you'll need to increase your activity level and/or muscle mass.

That said, a slow or damaged metabolism is rarely the cause of weight gain. It is "normal" to experience a slow-down of your metabolism as you age or become more sedentary, and to experience more physiological resistance to losing weight the leaner you get.

Bottom line: How much you eat, drink, and exercise, as well as your hormonal health, ultimately determine your weight.

WILL I LOSE MUSCLE?

Q: Will I lose muscle on the HCG Diet?

The research is very clear: when you diet and consume less calories in order to lose weight, your body is placed in a catabolic state. This means it breaks down tissue (muscle and fat) for its energy needs when there aren't enough calories present. For modern obesity treatments, the widely accepted guideline is about 25% muscle, and 75% fat but this varies with the individual and depends on a variety of factors which I discuss here. *

*Source: *https://www.ncbi.nlm.nih.gov/pmc/articles/PMC3970209/ Weight Loss Composition is One-Fourth Fat-Free Mass: A Critical Review and Critique of This Widely Cited Rule"*

Setting aside guidelines, the goal of any dieter shouldn't be just to lose weight but to *lose fat and preserve as much muscle as possible*. The smaller the calorie deficit, the less "catabolic" you become, so more lean muscle tissue is preserved when you only drop calories slightly. This is one reason experts recommend a slow and steady approach to weight loss: the standard is 1% of your body weight per week. In a 180-pound person, this is equal to 1.8 pounds per week. As you can see, a slow and steady weight loss of only 1% of your body weight per week can take a long time if you have a lot of weight to lose and being in a calorie deficit for months or even years can be difficult, mentally, and physically. This is one reason why the HCG Diet is so attractive: it might not be easy, but you can drop a lot of weight quickly.

Fast or Slow? Some people, like myself, are better designed physically and psychologically to lose weight in sprints and intervals than to approach fat loss as one big marathon. And let's face it: while a moderate and slow approach is best, there are also situations and life events that make rapid weight loss

> *desirable. It is also completely possible to*
> *maintain this loss provided you make the*
> *necessary nutrition and lifestyle changes. As I*
> *tell clients, "Diets can — and do — work, but*
> *they're temporary. They can get you to a certain*
> *point, but it's <u>habits</u> that keep you there."*

Other actions you can take to reduce muscle loss during a diet is to add in some form of resistance training, such as weight lifting, and to consume more protein. The Recommended Dietary Allowance (RDA) for protein is 0.8 grams of protein per kilogram of body weight (which is about .4 of a pound). In an 82-kilogram person (180-pound person), this is equivalent to about 70 grams of protein a day.

Keep in mind that the RDA is *the minimum* amount you need to prevent illness. New research suggests that this amount may be insufficient to promote optimal muscle health in all individuals.

> *The original Simeons Protocol only gives you*
> *about 45 grams of protein a day, which is*
> *another reason I no longer follow the Simeons*
> *Protocol.*

If you are active, dieting and/or restricting your carbohydrates, you should consume more protein as it has a muscle sparing effect. How much more? Well it depends on your activity levels and the protocol you're following.

In my opinion, HCG dieters should shoot for *at least* .5 grams of protein per pound body weight a day. I consumed over 100 grams of protein a day and still lost weight. If that sounds like a lot of protein, keep in mind that many people (especially the elderly) don't consume enough protein and over consume fats and carbs. This is especially true of the fat loss clients that I coach. Also note that most strength athletes consume 1 – 2 grams of protein per pound of body weight a day, with no ill effects.

As a person who weight trains 4x a week, losing muscle on the HCG Diet was of great concern to me, and not just because muscles make you strong and give you shape.

Muscles:

- allow a person to burn more calories at rest
- protect against osteoporosis
- protect against injury
- allow a person to live more independently (i.e., carry items)

I accept that muscle loss is inevitable during a diet, but I did everything I could to minimize it.

Why Losing Weight is Not as Important as Losing Fat

The more active you are, the better your "metabolism" is: you burn slightly more calories at rest due to greater muscle mass. You also burn calories working out, and even more calories just recovering from a workout. Muscles are a triple win.

This is why chronic yo-yo dieters can really struggle to lose weight and keep it off: a diet typically means losing fat as well as muscle tissue, and with more muscle lost through constant dieting, these individuals will burn fewer calories than someone who weighs the same but carries more muscle on their frame. Bottom line: the more sedentary you are, the less food you are able to eat without gaining weight. This is because your calorie needs are lower, and food that isn't burnt as fuel will be stored as fat.

If you strength train, you not only burn calories working out, you continue to burn a lot of calories throughout the day just recovering from a workout. This is because it takes a lot of fuel to repair muscle tissue and to refill those depleted glucose stores after a training session. In fact, you can burn calories for up to 48 hours after a workout: 100 or more a day, just recovering. This may not sound like much, but 100 calories a day just resting adds up to more than 10 pounds in a year, and that number doesn't include calories burnt through exercise. Just how important is exercise? According to long-range studies on obesity, people who have successfully lost weight and kept it off years later, almost always reported being "highly active".

Your focus, while dieting, should be to preserve as much muscle as you can. If you don't do some kind of weight training or resistance exercise while dieting, you will lose weight but a lot of what you lose may come from muscle as well as fat. Personally, I'd prefer to lose 21 pounds, and have 17 of it be fat and only 4 pounds be muscle, then lose 27 pounds and have 15 of it be fat and 12 pounds of it be muscle. Losing 27 pounds versus 21 pounds sounds more impressive, but it isn't particularly meaningful. This is why I prefer to focus on *fat* loss.

The Muscle Sparing Effects of HCG

So, muscle is good. And losing muscle is bad.

And since crash diets are supposed to make you lose a lot of muscle because your body essentially eats itself to lose weight, people think the HCG Diet is stupid.

Understandable.

Yet proponents of the HCG Diet claim the hormone has a muscle sparing effect. They say human chorionic gonadotropin hormone seems to "only" or "mostly", draw from fat stores and preserve lean muscle tissue, as long as people are using real HCG.

There is no research to support these claims, only anecdotal evidence, so where does this "muscle-preserving" claim come from?

Perhaps it is a marketing ploy to allay people's fears about following a rapid weight loss diet, which has been demonstrated to result in substantially greater muscle loss than a slower, more traditional approach. In one study, *subjects consumed a 500-calorie diet for 5 weeks while another group consumed 1200 calories a day for 12 weeks. The Fast Group lost 8x as much muscle mass as the Slow Group. * Interestingly, the subjects that lost more lean muscle mass also regained more bodyfat when the diet ended. Keep in mind, however, that these volunteers weren't taking HCG. Also, many weight-loss studies are done on obese, older, and/or sedentary populations so results may not be typical.*

Leaner individuals tend to lose more muscle on a diet, and the leaner you are, the more substantial this loss will be on a very low-calorie diet. Those who strength train, eat more protein, and carry more bodyfat generally experience less muscle loss while dieting.

---

*Source:
http://main.poliquingroup.com/ArticlesMultimedia/Articles/Article/27 16/Weight Loss Fast Or Slow Which Is Best.aspx "Weight Loss Fast or Slow: Which is Best?"

So, does the HCG hormone help preserve lean muscle mass while dieting? Perhaps. But I have it on good authority from someone who has treated hundreds of patients that it is a myth that the hormone "only" draws from fat stores and no muscle will be lost on the HCG Diet. Even a bodybuilder who eats a higher-protein, slightly higher-calorie diet (800 – 1000 calories) and continues to weight train can lose about 4% of her muscle mass on the HCG Diet. This is about half of what the sedentary volunteers lost in the 500-calorie study mentioned above.

So, how much muscle can you expect to lose on the HCG Diet if you're sedentary, don't train, and want to do the 500-calorie diet? Rayzel at HCGChica.com provides some excellent data on her blog. She lost 50 pounds over 5 rounds on the HCG diet. Rayzel followed the original Simeons Protocol and ate 500 calories (or less) a day. She eliminated the fruit and starches, and only exercised between diet rounds, as she found it too taxing to do CrossFit while consuming 500 calories a day.

Rayzel tracked her body composition with hydrostatic weighing and generously shares the results of those tests on her website at www.HCGChica.com. On Round 3, she lost 16.8 pounds of bodyfat and 4.2 pounds of muscle. This may sound minimal but it's actually quite typical for a diet. Based on these results, 25% of the weight that she lost was muscle, which is an industry acceptable guideline; fairly impressive given the severe protein and calorie restriction.

Based on these examples, it is possible the hormone does indeed have a slight muscle sparing effect, but the scientist in me requires more data before I can reach any conclusions. If you have any anecdotal evidence you can share with me, please email me at CoachingWithAdele@gmail.com.

Final Note: It's worth mentioning, that at the time of this

writing, Rayzel has also managed to keep the weight off for five years!

What Did Dr. Simeons Have to Say?

I think it's worth mentioning that when Dr. Simeons created his protocol, there was no way to accurately test bodyfat percentage and lean muscle mass in each patient. Which is why I'm unsure of claims that the HCG hormone has a muscle sparing effect compared to other diets. Although Dr. Simeons says the hormone targets "abnormal fat", nowhere in Dr. Simeons' book, *Pounds and Inches*, could I find anything referencing the muscle sparing effects of the hormone.

After all, the only way to determine how much muscle and fat a person has in their body is through one of our modern bodyfat testing methods, and some methods are more accurate than others. To determine exactly how much fat and muscle is lost from dieting, a test must be done before the diet begins, and again after it ends to compare the difference. The most accurate testing methods available are hydrostatic weighing and the DXA scan, which are hardly mainstream. The least accurate are bio-impedance scans and skinfold testing with calipers.

The DXA scan is so precise that I know exactly how much my right and left arm weighs, along with my legs and torso. I also know the percentage breakdown of bone, muscle, and fat. I can also track this information over time to see the effect each round of dieting has on my body.

To Recap: As a principle, you will lose muscle as well as fat anytime you lose weight. However, *how much* muscle you lose depends on:

1. How severely you restrict your calories.
2. How long you diet for (diets longer than 12 weeks result in a greater proportion of muscle loss).
3. How much protein you eat each day.
4. Whether you strength train during the diet.
5. What state your body is in when you begin a round (health, and if you have a recent history of dieting).
6. Your genetics. (Some people may be more catabolic.)
7. Your sex.
8. Your age.
9. How much extra fat you carry going into the diet.
10. Environmental factors like sleep. (Lack of sleep is more catabolic.)

As you can see, this is a complex subject.

The HCG hormone may have some role to play in reducing the amount of muscle that is lost on a very low-calorie diet, though to what degree I am unsure of at this time. Truly, more data is needed.

DOES THE DIET RESET YOUR METABOLISM?

Q: Does the HCG Diet reset your metabolism?

Dr. Simeons believed that obesity was caused not by overeating, but by a "diencephalic deficiency" which caused overeating. (The diencephalon is a part of the brain that plays several important roles in healthy brain and bodily function.) This certainly rings bells for me as I wonder if he was stumbling upon the concept of leptin resistance, before it was discovered almost 40 years later, in 1994.

Dr. Simeons believed that HCG therapy could remedy or repair the diencephalon, and therefore reset the metabolism, in effect, curing the root cause of obesity. Dr. Simeons even wrote that 60% - 70% of his cases experienced little or no difficulty in holding their weight permanently. This is a grey area, as I am not certain how long he kept in touch with his patients. Did he only see his patients when they came back for another round? Did they maintain after six months? A year? Five years? What amount of time qualifies as permanent?

Only a few studies have tracked successful dieters over the long-term to see how they maintained their loss and I am not aware of a single study that has tracked HCG Dieters specifically.

Many people claim the diet resets your brain chemistry and metabolism for permanent weight loss, but I feel this is more fiction than fact.

The good news is that through ongoing lifestyle modifications, people can and do maintain their weight-loss, or at least a good chunk of it

> *after a year. But without support, ongoing vigilance, and a conscious change in eating habits and lifestyle behaviors, the weight will come back.*

There are far too many people, including myself, who have done the original HCG Diet, only to regain all the weight they lost when they went back to their old eating patterns. The hard part isn't losing the weight; it's keeping it off.

CAN THE HCG DIET HELP TO CREATE A NEW WEIGHT SETPOINT?

Q: Does the HCG Diet help to create a new weight setpoint?

When people talk about resetting their metabolism, I suspect they are essentially talking about creating a new weight set point, from which they can comfortably maintain their new lower weight with ease. Can the HCG Diet help with this? Not really.

Once you lose weight, your body will want to rebound to previous weight levels. This is especially true if you have lost more than 10% of your bodyweight in one round. This is why I believe it's better to do shorter rounds, take a break, and work at the skills of maintaining your new weight before doing another round of HCG. This may also be why Dr. Simeons wouldn't allow his patients to lose more than 34 pounds at a time.

.caks also give your metabolism time to "reset" so you can begin again, anew. It's akin to filling up your gas tank so you can drive further.

Your body is in its most delicate state right after you finish a round, and this is why transitioning to normal eating should be done consciously and strategically. Ideally, you should use this time to develop new eating habits and lifestyle changes from which to maintain your new weight.

What this means is that there is no finish line when it comes to losing weight and keeping it off. It can take up to six months for your body to adapt and settle into to its new weight. The good news is, that if you maintain your new weight long enough, you can create a new "settling" point or "set" point, from which you can relax a little and enjoy a little looser eating without rebounding. However, you must remain vigilant. Weigh yourself daily, or at least every few days, and work on mastering some new eating habits.

Be kind to yourself: new habits take a long time to master. Because of this, you may regain some, or all your weight the first time you lose weight on the HCG Diet. You may even have to do another round of HCG. If you don't give up and keep incorporating new healthier habits and learning from your mistakes, you can be a successful "loser" in the long run.

Just understand that obesity is like having a monster that follows you around for life, and you will probably have to stay vigilant for the remainder of your days. If you consistently overeat and consume too many calories for your energy needs, you will gain all the weight back, and create possibly newer, higher weight set points for yourself.

I understand the struggle, but I also know that everyone has some personal challenge in life. It could be mental illness, it could be a disease, it could be an addiction to alcohol, or it could be obesity. We all face challenges. Finding ways to overcome our challenges provides us with our greatest life lessons and opportunities for personal growth.

Obesity might be a symptom of larger issues, such as mental health, trauma, loneliness, social isolation and even boredom or a lack of purpose in life. Some people need therapy or coaching for these issues. Most of all, they need the support of loved ones.

ISN'T IT RISKY TO DEVIATE FROM THE ORIGINAL HCG DIET?

Q: Isn't it risky to deviate from the original HCG Diet?

In his book, *Pounds and Inches,* Dr. Simeons states that "the slightest deviation from the diet has under HCG disastrous results as far as the weight is concerned". He talks about how consuming a single salted almond could cause weight gain:

> *Even seemingly insignificant deviations, particularly those that at first sight seem to be an improvement, are very liable to produce most disappointing results and even annul the effect completely. For instance, if the diet is increased from 500 to 600 or 700 Calories, the loss of weight is quite unsatisfactory.*
>
> - Dr. Simeons, *Pounds and Inches*

So, is this accurate?

Despite the fear-mongering, I was able to eat a lot of rogue foods and still lose a half a pound a day by consuming 1000+ calories a day, on average. Others, like me, have also gone "rogue" with different higher-calorie protocols and still lost significant amounts of weight.

So no, I don't believe this is true.

Of course, there are others who say that they have gained weight after eating only a little bit of something off-protocol. This seems to be more typical of those who restrict themselves to 500 calories or less. I am left wondering if the cheat was as small as they thought, and if there were more unconscious eating behaviors than they realized. I also wonder if the weight gain or stall was going to happen anyway, as stalls and gains during fat loss are quite normal – especially for women. Finally, eating so few calories can create more stress on the body and increase cortisol. When cortisol increases, there tends to be more water retention.

CAN I EAT MORE THAN 500 CALORIES AND STILL LOSE WEIGHT?

Q: Can I eat more than 500 calories and still lose lots of weight?

Absolutely! Having tried both the original Simeons Protocol and my own higher-calorie, high-protein diet I've nicknamed *The HCG Performance Diet*, I can say that I lost similar amounts of weight on both protocols (about a half-pound a day) but felt *much* better and had more energy when I averaged 1000 calories a day.

One of my clients, a woman in her late fifties, has also tried both protocols and lost similar amounts of weight. However, she reported having more energy on my protocol. On it, she consumed 800 - 1000 calories a day, and enjoyed a greater variety of foods, including a little chocolate every day. She lost 30 pounds in 60 days and went on to lose another 25 pounds in Round 2, for a total of 55 pounds. Her main activity was walking each day.

That's right: *fewer calories and stricter eating doesn't always equal more weight lost.* In fact, too few calories and nutrients can put you in shut down mode.

This is because of a phenomenon known as NEAT or Non-Exercise Activity Thermogenesis. When the body can't get enough fuel, it naturally tries to conserve energy by limiting movement, aka NEAT.

How Diet Effects NEAT

In science circles, all forms of movement that aren't categorized as sports-like exercise are considered NEAT (Non-Exercise Activity Thermogenesis). Examples include typing, walking to work, loading the dishwasher, and even fidgeting. NEAT is a key component in how we maintain, lose, or gain bodyfat. If you know someone with a "fast metabolism", it might just be that they move and fidget a lot more, or have a more active job, and thus burn several hundred more calories a day than you!

> *NEAT activities increase our metabolic rate and the cumulative impact of movement accounts for the vast majority of an individual's non-resting calorie needs.*

So, what happens when the body doesn't get enough calories from food? It starts to slow down in an effort to conserve energy.

Less Food = Less Movement

If you are normally quite active but catch yourself wanting to skip out on your workouts, take the elevator instead of the stairs, or park close to an entrance because you're too tired to walk across the parking lot, take it as a sign that you probably need to consume more food.

The less you move, the less calories you burn. Lack of movement not only reduces the number of calories burnt in a day – and that can be substantial – it can result in more muscle loss, lower your BMR (basal metabolic rate) and hinder your weight loss efforts.

The HCG Diet for Active People

There are HCG experts who advise limiting your physical activity to walking while on the HCG Diet. This is because vigorous exercise can create more hunger and cause people to go off protocol. It only makes sense: a 500-calorie diet may work for sedentary individuals, but it will be insufficient for highly active people. If your job requires a lot of physical labor, or you're an athlete, you will need to consume more than 500 calories a day. In fact, I don't think you'll have much of a choice in the matter: your body will let you know either through feelings of exhaustion or extreme hunger. This has nothing to do with willpower and everything to do with physiology.

As a woman who loves to lift heavy weights 3 - 4x a week, I learned this first-hand. I would feel physically exhausted during and after a workout until I bumped my calories and carbs. In fact, I "bonked" so hard on one weight workout that I had to run next door and get a Coke just to finish my set!

Research over the last six decades indicates that carbohydrates heavily influence athletic performance and recovery except in some very specific and unique cases.

Non-athletes and sedentary individuals won't feel the impact of extreme calorie reduction to the same degree as more active individuals.

WHY ARE FATS NOT ALLOWED ON THE DIET?

Q: Why are fats now allowed on the diet?

The general advice is to completely avoid fats while on the diet, since the hormone is supposed to make you very sensitive to fats. Personally, I would love to do an HCG round where I eat 1000 calories and include a lot of healthy fats. This would test my theory that *how much* you eat matters more than what you eat.

On a personal note, I have eaten 80 grams of fat in a day and actually lost 1.4 pounds the next day. A client of mine once ate a steak which contained 30 grams of fat. She still lost 1.3 pounds the next day and continued to shed weight all week. This is not to advocate a high-fat diet at all, but just to say that people may not be as sensitive to fats on the HCG Diet as is commonly believed.

The main reason to avoid fats, in my opinion, is because

they have more calories per gram and it is *very easy* to overconsume them. A gram of fat has 9 calories. A gram of carbohydrate or protein has only 4 calories.

Just how easy is it to go overboard with fats? A tablespoon of peanut butter, which, if properly measured on a measuring spoon and levelled off and not rounded, is a much smaller serving than most people realize. A mere tablespoon of peanut butter contains a whopping 100 calories: lick it, and it's gone. On the other hand, a small apple is about 80 calories and a lot more filling – just try to eat three apples! When you're on a diet, it's vital to your success to find foods that are filling but low in calories and high in nutrients to keep you feeling satisfied and in the best possible state of health.

Interestingly enough, some HCG protocols recommend 1 – 2 tablespoons of coconut oil every day. This may fly in the face of the original protocol but somehow, people still manage to lose weight…

Diets work because they keep you in a caloric deficit. It doesn't matter if it's ketogenic, vegan, Atkins, low-carb, low-fat, flexible dieting or Nutrisystem. In fact, a low-fat, moderate carb diet has proven just as successful as a high-fat, low-carb diet. *

If you can manage your hunger and consume less, you will lose weight (as long as you're in good health and good hormonal shape). However, some people find certain approaches are more satisfying and pleasant for them personally and yield better results than other approaches. But at the end of the day, the best diet is the diet you can stick with to achieve the results you desire.

---

*Source: *https://www.ncbi.nlm.nih.gov/pmc/articles/PMC2763382/*
"Reduced-calorie diets result in clinically meaningful weight loss regardless of which macronutrients they emphasize."

CAN I DIET FOR LESS THAN THREE WEEKS?

Q: I only want to lose a little weight. Can I diet for less than three weeks?

Rounds shorter than 26 days are not advised. According to Dr. Simeons in *Pounds and Inches,* "We never give a treatment lasting less than 26 days, even in patients needing to lose only 5 pounds. It seems that even in the mildest cases of obesity the diencephalon requires about three weeks rest from the maximal exertion to which it has been previously subjected in order to regain fully its normal fat-banking capacity."

Translation: Don't come off the medication sooner than 23 days. The 26 days is equal to 2 days of Phase 1 loading with the medication, plus 21 days of Phase 2 dieting with the medication, plus 3 days of Phase 3 dieting with no medication. Dr. Simeons advises losing the weight, then slightly increasing your calories just enough to maintain your weight loss (he suggested 800 calories for maintenance). Then stop the medication after 23 days and continue to eat at maintenance for three more days to give your body a chance to flush out the HCG. Otherwise, the risk of regaining is much higher (apparently).

So, is this accurate?

On a personal and somewhat related note, I terminated a round early due to hunger from *too much* HCG hormone in my body: I was only on the diet for two weeks. During those two weeks, I gained six pounds during the preload and only lost six pounds in Phase 2 (I was constantly overeating while taking the hormone, which is probably worse than ending a round early). Although I stopped taking the medication well before the 23 days were over, I returned to my starting weight and maintained it within a few pounds. This should be a comfort to anyone who has to terminate a round early.

WHERE WILL I LOSE THE MOST FAT?

Q: Where will I lose the fat?

You will lose fat all over your body: face, belly, arms, legs and back – even the neck and ankles – but you may find some areas shrink more visibly than others and it won't be "even". Nor should you expect stubborn areas of fat to quickly melt away, despite popular claims.

Based on my own personal experience, stubborn areas take longer to lose.

Since a DXA scan measures every inch of your body from head to toe, I could track my muscle and fat loss over time. I knew precisely how much each of my limbs and torso weighed, and the percentage breakdown of fat and muscle lost over time. I even knew my intra-abdominal or visceral fat, the most dangerous kind of fat to have since it secretes a protein known to increase resistance to insulin. High visceral fat has been linked to cancer, stroke, Alzheimer's disease, and dementia.

After my second round, I discovered I lost comparatively little fat around and, in my belly, and yet, this is where I had the most to lose! My legs had been the leanest part of me, and yet I lost the most fat, percentage-wise, in my legs. This was a little disappointing as I really wanted to lose the belly, which had reduced, but not as much as I'd have liked. Another round of HCG would hopefully address that stubborn area in the future.

CAN I TAKE HCG WHILE MENSTRUATING?

Q: Can I take HCG while menstruating?

Dr. Simeons advised stopping injections when menstruation began, and resuming them as soon as menstruation ended. He observed that patients became extremely hungry unless the injections resumed at once.

From his book, *Pounds and Inches*, "In menstruating women, the best time to start treatment is immediately after a period. Treatment may also be started later, but it is advisable to have at least ten days in hand before the onset of the next period. Similarly, the end of a course should never be made to coincide with onset of menstruation."

Some people continue to follow this advice; others do not. Some stop taking medication only on their heaviest flow days, and others take it throughout.

Is HCG basically just an appetite suppressant?

Q: Is HCG basically just an appetite suppressant?

I think HCG does more than just suppress the appetite: it also seems to impact and regulate the hormones (See the section: Will the HCG Diet mess up my hormones?). However, my approach to the HCG Diet is that the hormone is essentially an appetite suppressant, one that works better and has fewer side effects than anything I've tried in the past.

Like many people who have struggled to lose weight, I've tried various appetite suppressants including over-the-counter supplements and even a doctor-prescribed diet pill that I stopped taking due to lack of results and too many negative side effects. It had a stimulating effect and caused insomnia and sweating. In fact, any diet pill or medicine I've tried in the past has been a waste of money and a disappointment.

On the HCG medication, I experienced almost no negative side effects. If anything, it seemed to increase my mental clarity, my hot flashes disappeared, and I felt very "even keel" physically. It was like having a lot of really good days strung together. If I experienced an energy crash, it was always the result of too few calories or carbs.

WILL THE HCG DIET MESS UP MY HORMONES?

Q: Will the HCG Diet mess up my hormones?

It is unlikely but not impossible. (If anything, my hormones seemed to benefit from HCG.) Here, I think it's important to distinguish between the Diet, and the Hormone itself, and how each may impact our body.

The Diet: We do know that testosterone, leptin, and thyroid hormones tend to decrease the longer you stay in a caloric deficit *on any diet*. The more severe the calorie restriction, the more impact there is on our hormones, especially the thyroid. However, the HCG hormone may play a protective role in limiting that damage.

The Hormone: Dr. Simeons believed that the HCG hormone could remedy a dysfunctional hypothalamus, which, he believed, was the root cause of obesity. He also would have his patients stop taking thyroid medication during the course of injections. Since the hypothalamus is a master gland that regulates thyroid function, I find it interesting that there are studies indicating that human chorionic gonadotropin hormone can actually help stimulate thyroid function and increase thyroid hormone release. * I believe Dr. Simeons was onto something here, and it is worthy of more research.

*Source: _https://www.ncbi.nlm.nih.gov/pubmed/1648698_ and _https://www.ncbi.nlm.nih.gov/pubmed/8045981_

> I have hypothyroidism (Hashimoto's Thyroiditis) and I've taken medication for it for 30 years. My thyroid labs actually improved and looked better than they ever had before, when I had my TSH, T3, T4 and antibodies tested in Round 2.
>
> And on the topic of menopause: my hot flashes and night sweats completely disappeared while taking the medication, only to resume when I stopped. Furthermore, I have become very temperature sensitive in the last couple of years. I can become very cold or very hot within a few degrees. While I was on the HCG, I felt very even keel, like my body was better able to thermoregulate.
>
> This experience repeated at every round. It was a completely unexpected but welcome side benefit of the medication. To be honest, I have come to miss how good and 'stable' the HCG made me feel.*.

Interestingly enough, I had to decrease my thyroid dosage by 25% in the last few days of Round 2, and continued to reduce it when the diet ended, only upping it slightly after six months had passed. Being on an ultra-low-calorie diet should have theoretically lowered my thyroid, but the HCG hormone seemed to have stimulated it. This may be due to the following reasons:

1. The HCG hormone does improve hypothalamus and/or thyroid function as Dr. Simeons states;

2. I may have needed less medication because I was now a smaller person.

More research is needed.

Bottom line, if you take thyroid medication, you may need to adjust your dose either during or after you lose weight on the HCG Diet. Discuss your concerns with your physician.

IS IT TRUE YOU WILL TEST POSITIVE FOR PREGNANCY ON THE HCG HORMONE?

Q: Is it true you will test positive for pregnancy on the HCG hormone?

Since pregnancy tests are designed to detect human chorionic gonadotropin in the urine, I was curious to see if I would test positive for pregnancy while taking HCG. I purchased several over-the-counter pregnancy tests and ran a urine test while on the homeopathic drops, pellets, and injections. Each time, the result was negative. This is probably due to the fact that a pregnant woman excretes much more HCG hormone than dieters do.

I then ran the same experiment a second time, but this time I applied the product *directly* to the pregnancy kit.

I recorded the entire experiment in a series of short videos on YouTube. (If you subscribe to my mailing list at TheHCGDietBook.com, you'll receive a link to the videos.)

Here are the results:

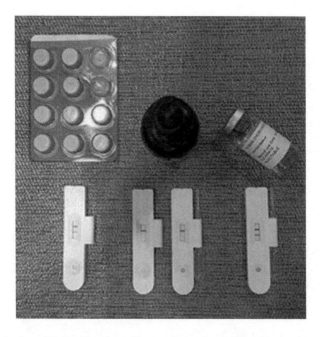

Left to Right: Troches, Drops, Injections. The drops were tested twice and both tests yielded a negative result. The troches (pills) and injections tested positive.

1. Homeopathic drops – I used a fresh, unopened bottle to ensure potency and placed a few drops on a pregnancy kit. The result was negative (no HCG detected). According to the manufacturer, the homeopathic drops were supposed to contain the equivalent of 125 IU of HCG per 30 drops. Just in case the concentration was too low, I did a second test, and added more drops but that test was also negative. I believe a lack of HCG was the reason I was so hungry on the drops compared to the pellets and injections.

2. HCG oral troches – I mixed the pills I got from DietDoc.com with some bacteriostatic water and then placed a few drops of liquid on the pregnancy test. The result was positive for HCG.

3. HCG injections – After mixing the HCG powder and bacteriostatic water in a vial, I filled a syringe and placed a few drops on a pregnancy test. The result was also positive for HCG.

WILL I FEEL WEAK AND TIRED?

Q: Will I feel weak and tired?

I felt weak on a 500-calorie diet and just walking around a grocery store could wear me out. As soon as I increased my calories and carbs, I felt great: I could strength train 4x a week (not quite as heavy of course), walk daily, and hike on weekends, and still have energy left over. Finding that sweet spot can take a bit of experimentation because everyone is unique. Personally, I feel much better with a higher-calorie, higher-protein, non-ketogenic and carb-timed approach to fat loss.

Not everyone feels horrible on 500 calories, but many people will. And if you have thyroid issues, you may not be a suitable candidate for a low-carb diet. Always listen to your body.

Note: The first 3 - 5 days of the diet are the toughest as your body adjusts to less carbs and sugar and you may feel more tired than usual. It's also my understanding that it takes time for the hormone to reach maximum effect in the body. Day 5, for me, was always the hardest and hungriest. I recommend starting the very low-calorie part of the diet when you don't have a lot of demands.

WILL I HAVE BRAIN FOG?

Q: Will I have brain fog, and trouble concentrating?

When I tried a ketogenic version of the HCG Diet, I experienced a bit of brain fog in the first week.

Otherwise, I was mentally alert and brimming with ideas every time I did a round with prescription HCG. I could focus for hours. I even researched and wrote much of this book while I was dieting.

WILL I SLEEP OKAY?

Q: Will I sleep okay?

Other than the first few days and the last few days of the diet (on each round), I slept very well for the most part, averaging 8 - 9 hours a night with no night sweats.

Having counted macros in the past, I know that when I consume less than 150 grams of carbohydrates I typically have difficulty sleeping and will wake up during the night. However, I had no such issues on the HCG Diet even though I averaged less than 100 grams of carbohydrates a day.

There were a couple times I woke up during the night because I felt hot; I threw off the covers while my husband stayed nestled under the quilt. I believe this is because my metabolism was revving, and not because of menopause. As I mentioned, I never experienced hot flashes while taking the medication, and this was an unexpected but welcome benefit.

Some people do get insomnia on the diet. This may be due to hunger or simply insufficient calories. I recommend having a casein protein shake (mixed with water, not milk) or some plain fat-free Greek yogurt or cottage cheese before bed. The extra calories and the tryptophan from the dairy may help you sleep. Of course, this is not part of the original Simeons Protocol but if you don't mind going off-plan and having dairy, it's worth a try. In my opinion, a lack of sleep has the potential to derail your diet more than 150 calories.

A bad day almost always results from a

crappy night of sleep. If I don't get eight hours of rest, I crave sweets and carbs, my mood plummets, I lose my motivation to exercise, and I find it hard to focus. Basically, I am on system shutdown. Insufficient sleep is the surest way to sabotage my weight-loss efforts. I now prioritize sleep above everything else because it effects everything else.

From my book, Forty Daze:
A Quest for Self-Improvement

Casein protein is a slow-digesting protein that forms a bolus in your stomach and takes a lot of time to metabolize. Because of this, it provides a trickle of amino acids to your muscles and tissues while you sleep. The amino acids help preserve, repair, and build lean muscle tissue while you sleep. It is filling, and it's the ideal protein to have before bedtime (unless you are lactose intolerant.)

Whey protein has a much faster release rate, which makes it better for right after a workout when your muscles are "thirsty" and could benefit from a full blast of amino acids.

I use Optimum Nutrition's Gold Standard 100% Casein. It comes in vanilla and a variety of flavors like Cookies and Cream and Peanut Butter. I prefer to mix it with a tiny bit of water and chill it for half an hour, so it forms a pudding-like texture. I will also mix it with water and baking powder and bake a couple "cookies" in the toaster oven and enjoy them with a glass of unsweetened almond milk before bed.

SHOULD I TAKE VITAMINS?

Q: Should I take vitamins on the HCG Diet?

Some protocols don't recommend them, while others do. I believe they are beneficial while dieting, though you should always consult with your doctor and pharmacist. Your doctor will tell you what vitamins are appropriate for you to consume, and your pharmacist will tell you if certain vitamins may interact with your medication.

The science on multivitamins as a preventative for disease is inconclusive according to the National Institute of Health. However, most dieticians recommend a multivitamin and fish oil/omega-3 fatty acid supplementation for the prevention of heart disease. Look at your lab work and discuss any concerns, along with any vitamin deficiencies with your physician. You may benefit from supplementation.

While on the diet, I continued to take my normal supplements each day. This included 3000 IU of Vitamin D3 (I'm deficient, according to my bloodwork), 400 mg of magnesium, a high-potency woman's multivitamin, 100 mcg selenium (for thyroid), and the occasional fish oil tablet (when I could remember). For the HCG Diet in particular, I added 99 mg of potassium and 1000 mg of sublingual B12 during Phase 2 and 3. I continued taking my thyroid medication throughout.

One of the reasons so many people are against the HCG Diet is that an ultra-low-calorie diet often results in a lack of vitamins and nutrients. This, in turn, can cause electrolyte imbalances, cramping, headaches, and in rare cases, an irregular heartbeat. To mitigate this, some HCG'ers take electrolytes, and/or daily potassium, along with a multivitamin while on the diet. People have also experienced hair loss from multiple or extended diet rounds, in which case, some people recommend taking biotin. However, there is insufficient evidence to support the use of biotin as an effective treatment for hair loss and the hair loss may be due to other factors.

Many HCG Diet doctors also offer B12 injections to help patients with flagging energy.

Stay away from gummy vitamins and added sugars in your vitamins. If you have Hashimotos thyroiditis, you may wish to avoid supplements that contain soy.

The Sufficient Vitamin Myth

One thing that has always struck me as peculiar is the notion that as your body burns up its fat stores, stored vitamins and nutrients will be released back into the body in sufficient amounts for the body's health.

> *"Sooner or later most patients express a fear that they may be running out of vitamins or that the restricted diet may make them anemic. On this score the physician can confidently relieve their apprehension by explaining that every time they lose a pound of fatty tissue, which they do almost daily, only the actual fat is burned up;* **all the vitamins, the proteins, the blood, and the minerals which this tissue contains in abundance are fed back into the body.**
>
> -   Dr. Simeons, *Pounds and Inches*

This is only partly true. Some nutrients like **proteins and water-soluble vitamins cannot be stored in the body.** However, fat-soluble vitamins, hormones, and pollutants are all stored in the liver and fatty tissue.

> *Water-soluble vitamins include Vitamins B1, B2, B3, B5, B6, B7, B9, B12 and C. Except for B6 and B12, water-soluble vitamins cannot be stored in the body and are excreted in the urine. As a result, these vitamins must be consumed through a variety*

of food sources and/or supplementation.

Fat-soluble vitamins include Vitamins A, D, E, and K are often found in fat-containing foods. Unlike water-soluble vitamins, fat-soluble vitamins can be stored in the body for long periods of time and are excreted in the feces. However, fats aren't permitted on the HCG Diet, so it is impossible to ensure adequate amounts are being met over the duration of the diet.

As you lose weight, the fat cells shrink and release lipids (for energy), as well as stored nutrients and toxins back into your bloodstream. These get broken down further and exit your body through your breath and urine.

If "all the vitamins, the proteins, the blood, and the minerals" are fed back into the body when the fat is burned up, why would we need to consume additional vitamins and give people B12 shots? Because the amounts are insufficient. This idea also assumes individuals ate well enough prior to dieting, so that they had sufficient amounts of vitamins stored in their fatty tissue. In this modern age of highly processed food, people may be obese, but still starved for adequate amounts of nutrients and vitamins.

Essential Amino Acids

While some vitamins are recycled back into the bloodstream, essential amino acids cannot be manufactured or stored in the body and must be consumed daily in sufficient amounts from outside sources. ("Essential" means necessary for function.) Fish, meat, and eggs have the highest concentration of essential amino acids. *

Source: _https://www.symptomfind.com/nutrition-supplements/essential-amino-acids_

Our knowledge of nutrition and the importance of protein has greatly advanced over the last several decades. Unfortunately, many people still adhere to the original Simeons Protocol, which doesn't even come close to meeting the minimum RDA (Recommended Daily Allowance) of protein and essential nutrients per day.

WHY IS PROTEIN SO IMPORTANT?

Q: Why is protein so Important?

Protein is the building block of tissue in your body. Every cell has protein as part of its makeup. Protein helps:

- Grow and repair tissue
- Build muscle
- Heal injuries
- Strengthen the immune system
- Synthesize hormones

…And more.

Protein also increases satiety, which means it increases a

sense of fullness, which is helpful during a diet as well as during maintenance.

IS THE MEAL PLAN HARD TO FOLLOW?

Q: Is the meal plan and diet hard to follow?

Preparing your meals and following the diet is dead simple. The hard part is staying disciplined and committed through all four phases, and to the protocol you choose. As they say, "Simple, but not easy." The good thing is, you don't have to diet for very long to lose a substantial amount of weight.

The food itself is very straight forward, and you'll save lots of time preparing and cooking your meals and cleaning up afterwards. (Unless you love to cook and want to experiment with different HCG Diet recipes.)

One thing I ate every week was a frittata. I'd bake up a carton of egg whites with spinach, tomatoes and mushrooms in the oven and it would last me for 4 meals. Every couple of weeks, I'd make turkey spaghetti sauce in the crockpot and freeze half of it. This would yield about 8 meals and I'd eat the spaghetti sauce over miracle noodles for a hearty low-carb meal of "spaghetti". I'd also cook up some chicken breasts and keep them in the fridge to throw in a salad with some 0-calorie dressing. It was all very simple and easy – much easier than "real" life! The hardest part of the diet is eating out and I recommend avoiding restaurants as much as possible while you're in Phase 2.

If you like to cook and/or variety is important to you, I recommend googling "Free HCG Diet recipes" for meal ideas.

WHAT IF I'M NOT HUNGRY AT ALL?

Q: What if I'm not hungry at all?

Some people completely lose their appetite with the hormone, and just the thought of eating makes them want to gag. They could happily survive on 250 calories a day. Dr. Simeons said a lack of appetite and inability to eat is a "not uncommon experience". In that case, he advised skipping the second meal on Phase 2, Day 1. However, he didn't elaborate on what to do if a lack of hunger continues past Day 1.

The prevailing wisdom for followers of the Simeons Protocol is that it is fine to miss a meal or skip some food items if you aren't hungry, but I advise against it because your body needs the vitamins, nutrients, and electrolytes to function properly. Also, eating too few calories can slow or stall your weight-loss efforts.

People (including myself) have lost as much, or even more weight, consuming 800+ calories a day as they do eating 500 or fewer calories.

If eating feels *impossible*, then I recommend only skipping your starches like the melba toast or bread sticks, which have little nutritional value. In order of importance, I always prioritize protein, then vegetables, then fruit, then starches. I do not recommend ever skipping the protein. If choking down some egg whites or chicken breast is revolting, consider some plain, fat-free Greek yogurt or cottage cheese mixed with stevia and cinnamon, or a low-carb, zero fat, zero sugar protein shake.

I'M VEGETARIAN. CAN I DO THE HCG DIET?

Q: I'm Vegetarian. Can I do this diet?

Vegans will have a tough time on the original HCG Diet. I don't recommend it, unless you are willing to make exceptions, and consume things like milk, egg whites, and protein powders as your protein sources. As Dr. Simeons states in his book, "Strict vegetarians such as orthodox Hindus present a special problem, because milk and curds are the only animal protein they will eat. To supply them with sufficient protein of animal origin they must drink 500 cc. of skimmed milk per day, though part of this ration can be taken as curds. As far as fruit, vegetables and starch are concerned, their diet is the same as that of nonvegetarians; they cannot be allowed their usual intake of vegetable proteins from leguminous plants such as beans or from wheat or nuts, nor can they have their customary rice. In spite of these severe restrictions, their average loss is about half that of non-vegetarians, presumably owing to the sugar content of the milk."

That said, some people have had success with a vegan approach. I recommend forums such as HCGDietInfo.com for more information.

How important is Phase 1?

Q: I can eat a lot, but I don't want to binge. How important is it to eat a lot of food in Phase 1? What if I'm not that hungry?

If you'll recall, Phase 1 is the Pre-Diet or Loading Phase of any protocol. This is where you eat to capacity for two to three days while taking your HCG medication. It is extremely important to eat as much as possible *without making yourself sick* during this time. This helps to rev up your metabolism for the next phase and (reportedly) helps to minimize cravings and hunger in the first week of Phase 2.

It sounds counter-intuitive: "Eat to lose!" but it works. The people who seem to have the most success eat to capacity in Phase 1. They follow the diet, and the diet, ironically, starts with Phase 1 – gorging.

If you are resisting this idea of gaining weight in Phase 1, or eating when you're not hungry, consider that it's only two to three days but it will affect your entire round. Be as disciplined about this phase as you would be about Phase 2.

> *I did a 2-day load once where I didn't eat a lot because I wasn't hungry. I experienced much better results when I did a 3-day dirty load and ate to the point of discomfort. It got to the point where food disgusted me. That's pretty much how you want to feel at the end of your loading phase: like you just finished Thanksgiving Dinner and you don't want another bite.*

The truth is, the HCG hormone may start to kick in as quickly as Day 2, and it may feel like you're forcing food into your mouth. Try to eat every two hours, even if you have to set an alarm on your phone to remind yourself. Just don't get up in the middle of the night to eat: get your normal amount of sleep and eat throughout the day.

If you're doing a dirty load, feel free to eat anything you like, barring any food allergies or medical issues. Your choices don't have to be completely unhealthy: you can still have a salad, just make sure you have lots of fats with it: nuts, cheese, oils, avocado, and croutons can push a salad over 1000 calories. That's a good meal for Phase 1. If you're struggling to get the food down, consider liquid calories like olive oil, milkshakes, bubble tea, and smoothies. You could also do more soft foods like ice-cream, rice pudding, nut butters, avocado and brie cheese. The general rule of thumb is to prioritize fats in Phase 1. The extra fats are believed to help spread the HCG hormone throughout the body, though I can find no evidence to support this claim.

I made a list of all the food I wanted to eat in Round 3, Phase 1, and I'm glad I did. I lost my appetite and it served as a checklist. I would eat something and cross it off, methodically working my way down the list.

You are on this diet because you gained weight, likely due to overeating: why be stubborn about not overeating now?

If you are doing a dirty load, you can expect to gain 5 - 10 pounds, but that weight will come off in the first two to three days of Phase 2. If you are doing a dirty load and haven't gained at least four pounds after two days, make sure you do a third day of loading. If you have been dieting or undereating prior to starting the HCG Diet, it is especially important to do a three-day load as you will be in a depleted state. Dr. Simeons used to have patients load up for an entire week if they were in poor condition before starting the HCG Diet!

> *Patients whose general condition is low, owing to excessive previous dieting, must eat to capacity for about one week before starting treatment, regardless of how much weight they may gain in the process. One cannot keep a patient comfortably on 500 Calories unless his normal fat reserves are reasonably well stocked. It is for this reason also that every case, even those that are actually gaining must eat to capacity of the most fattening food they can get down until they have had the third injection. It*

*is a fundamental mistake to put a patient on
500 Calories as soon as the injections are
started, as it seems to take about three
injections before abnormally deposited fat
begins to circulate and thus become available.*

- Dr. Simeons, *Pounds and Inches*

WILL I GAIN THE WEIGHT BACK?

Q: Will I gain all the weight back once the diet is over?

You will gain the weight back if you:

1. Eat more calories than your body requires.

2. Don't address any undiagnosed/untreated hormonal issues or food sensitivities/allergies that may be affecting your health.

3. Take action as soon as you gain more than a few pounds.

The general consensus is that it is imperative to stay away from sugar and starches during the 3-week transition in Phase 3 (which I refer to as Phase 4). Personally, I've enjoyed toast with jam and other prohibited starchy and sugary items in this three-week phase, but I ate *very little* of them. As a result, I was still able to maintain my loss.

So where does this information come from? I believe any weight gain is mainly caused by overwhelming and overloading your glycogen stores, *especially* if you are coming off a keto-based diet. Furthermore, it is very easy to overeat such highly palatable foods and trigger cravings for more sugary, starchy foods. A good rule of thumb for Phase 4 is to just eat more of the same kind of foods you ate in Phase 2, but add more variety when it comes to fruits, vegetables, healthy fats, and lean proteins.

Muscle versus Fat

If you're an active gym-goer, there is no need to freak out if you gain a little weight. Chances are, you're putting on muscle, and that's a good thing. For example, if you lift weights at least three times a week, and push yourself in the gym, you can expect to gain as much as 5 – 20 pounds in your first year of lifting (on the lower end for females and the higher end for males). This should not be mistaken for fat.

If you lift weights regularly, try not to gain more than 1% of your bodyweight a month (if you're in a massing or gaining phase, try to limit this to 0.5% a week) or you may be putting on more fat than muscle.

This is why taking body measurements can be so valuable: if the inches on the tape measure stay the same or go down, you are losing fat, even if the scale goes up. Trying to judge things based on how your clothes fit is not a good gauge: if you wear leggings or loose clothes, you can easily pack on ten pounds without a visible difference.

A bodyfat analysis can be very useful for keeping track of your bodyfat and muscle mass over time.

COMPARING BODY FAT TESTING METHODS

Q: What methods exist to test your bodyfat?

In order of accuracy from the most accurate to least accurate:

1. DXA scan (Dual-energy X-ray Absorptiometry)
2. Hydrostatic weighing (dunk tank)
3. Air displacement plethysmography (bod pod)
4. Bioelectrical Impedance
5. Callipers skinfold measurements

HOW IS A DXA SCAN DONE?

Q: How is a DXA scan done?

Essentially, you lay on a table and a machine scans you from head to toe with your clothes on (no metal allowed). It takes about ten minutes and the amount of radiation is negligible. A DXA scan is the most precise way to measure how much bone, fat, and muscle you have in your body. It is accurate within 3%.

HOW DOES A DXA SCAN COMPARE TO OTHER TYPES OF BODY FAT TESTING?

Q: How does a DXA Scan compare to other types of body fat testing?

A DXA scan tends to show higher body fat results than other methods but it is widely believed to be the most consistent and most precise of all methods. This is because every inch of your body is scanned, and all of your tissues are analyzed: bone, muscle, and fat are all calculated to a very precise degree. Bonus: A DXA scan will also tell you your bone mass as well as your lean muscle mass and fat percentage in each limb, and even your intraabdominal fat, which is the most dangerous type of fat to have. I'm not aware of any other method that can do this.

HAS ANYONE EVER COMPARED THE DIFFERENT BODYFAT TESTS, ON THE SAME INDIVIDUAL, ALL IN THE SAME MORNING?

Q: Has anyone ever compared the different bodyfat tests, on the same individual, all in the same morning?

Yes! Check out *The Big Fat Experiment* and learn just how wildly different the results can be:
https://www.bodyspec.com/blog/post/the_big_fat_experiment

In summary, Elaine is 5'3" and 130 pounds. She trains twice a week at powerlifting and does Pilates. She had her body fat measured five different ways, all in the same morning. Her bioelectric impedance scale indicated she was 24.6% bodyfat, her BodPod said she was 22.3%

bodyfat, her DXA scan said she was 27% bodyfat, her caliper tests said she was anywhere from 22% - 25%, and her hydrostatic dunk tank said she was only 19.8% body fat. That's a difference of 7.2% between the hydrostatic dunk tank and the DXA scan!

HOW MUCH DOES A DXA SCAN COST?

Q: How much does a DXA scan cost?

A DXA scan can cost $400 at a hospital but is normally $45 - $100 at a private clinic. I used BodySpec in Los Angeles for all my appointments and paid $45 a session.

ANY OTHER TIPS FOR CALCULATING MY BODYFAT AND LEAN MUSCLE?

Q: Any other tips for calculating my bodyfat and lean muscle?

Whatever method you choose, it is best to stick with the same one in order to track your progress over time because different methods yield different results. For example, Elaine's hydrostatic test results in *The Big Fat Experiment* said she was 19.8% bodyfat. However, her DXA scan indicated 27% bodyfat. These tests were performed in the same morning. Similarly, my DXA scan indicated my bodyfat was 32.5% but the handheld bio-impedance device at my gym indicated 27% bodyfat: a

5.5% variation. I did both tests within an hour of each other and didn't consume any food or drink between tests. As you can see, jumping from method to method will make it impossible to accurately track your progress.

DON'T BODYFAT TESTING RESULTS VARY BASED ON THE EQUIPMENT, YOUR HYDRATION LEVELS, ETC.?

Q: Don't bodyfat testing results vary a lot based on the equipment, what you drink, eat, user error, etc.

Yes, they can! So whatever method you use to track your progress, it's always best to try to keep your conditions roughly the same. That means you would ideally test yourself with the same person, device, or machine, at the same time of day each time, eating and drinking the same things, and wearing the same clothes at each appointment. Exercise can also affect your scores, so I chose not to exercise the morning before my tests.

Will drinking water affect my bodyfat results?

Yes, but to what degree depends on the testing device. Bioelectrical impedance devices are very sensitive to hydration levels when giving a body fat percentage result, but DXA scans aren't.

To prove this, Jason, the co-founder of BodySpec, had a scan done, then chugged an entire gallon of water. He had a second scan done before running off to the men's room. The result? His bodyfat went down by a measly pound.

(By the way, a gallon of water is *a lot* of water. It is equal to 16 glasses and weighs a little over eight pounds.)

Even more interesting, his lean tissue went up by 7.4 pounds. Yes, Jason seemingly gained more than seven pounds of lean muscle tissue just by saturating his muscles with water.

Can you see how easy it is to manipulate the result of a person's bodyfat percentage and lean muscle mass, even using something as precise as a DXA scan?

To read the full story, visit - https://www.bodyspec.com/blog/post/will_drinking_water_affect_my_scan

WHAT IF THE TEST SAYS I'M OBESE OR OVERWEIGHT, BUT I DON'T AGREE?

Q: What if the test says I'm obese or overweight, but I don't agree?

I didn't agree with my results either! However, numbers don't lie. 32.5% is 32.5%. The problem is in how we interpret these numbers.

Medical and fitness professionals use a range of bodyfat percentages to classify people as underweight", "normal", "overweight" or "obese", and I believe these ranges are based on the most popular (and not necessarily accurate) methods of measuring bodyfat.

For example, I was 32.5% bodyfat according to my DXA scan. I was 27% bodyfat according to a bioelectrical impedance test taken at my gym that same morning. DXA scans are not popular but bioelectrical impedance devices are because they're inexpensive.

According to the medical classifications, I am obese based on the results of my DXA scan, and normal based on the results of my bioelectrical impedance test.

So, what is true? Well, I believe I am 32.5% bodyfat, but I am definitely not obese. The DXA scan may be more accurate, but the 27% reading I got from the bioelectrical impedance test puts me in a more appropriate category.

It may be time for medical and fitness professionals to adjust the bodyfat ranges for what is considered "overweight" versus "obese" versus "normal" based on the different methods available. If a person tests with hydrostatic weighing and their number is off by 7% from a DXA scan, then different categories should exist for the different methods. Otherwise, it's all a bit meaningless.

> *When I see a YouTube or Instagram bodybuilder say he's 5% body fat, my first thought is: what method did he use to test himself?*

The main takeaway is to use your body fat tests, your scale, and your measuring tape as *tools* to extract data from. They are merely numbers to help you gauge your progress over time.

After all, the goal shouldn't be to just lose weight: the goal should be to lose fat and preserve or increase your muscle.

Are you seeing changes in body fat over time? If your scale goes up, but your body fat test shows you have dropped fat and gained muscle, then things are heading in a great direction!

Despite popular claims, a pound of fat weighs exactly the same as a pound of muscle: they both weigh a pound. They just take up different amounts of space in your body; fat takes up more volume.

Don't get too hung up about the number on the bodyweight scale: it cannot tell you how fit you are. Have a look at 180 pounds, 5'7" pro strong woman Brittany Diamond on Instagram. She is a strong, curvy Amazon woman who blows away expectations of what a 180-pound woman looks like.

BODY FAT CLASSIFICATIONS FOR MEN AND WOMEN

Q: What are the body fat classifications for men and women?

Essential bodyfat:

Men: 2 – 4%

Women: 9 – 11%

Underweight or Athletic:

Men: 6 – 13%

Women: 14 – 20%

Fit:

Men: 14 – 17%

Women: 21 – 24%

Normal:

Men: 18 – 25%

Women: 25 – 31%

Overweight/Obese:

Men: 26%+

Women: 32%+

- Essential bodyfat is exactly what it says: the fat needed to function properly. It includes padding around the eyeballs and organs, and in the heels of your feet so you can walk.
- Underweight or Athletic ranges look fit. At the lower ranges they look "ripped" or "shredded" like a bodybuilder. At the lowest ranges, menstruation stops in women.

- Fit ranges look heathy, (many college students fall into this range), but not "shredded" like an athlete.
- The middle range of "Normal" starts to look overweight.
- Health problems occur in the obese range.

These classifications are likely not based on DXA scans.

*Source of chart: *"How to Calculate Your Body Fat Percentage Easily & Accurately"* at https://legionathletics.com/how-to-calculate-body-fat

WHAT IF I HAVE TO TRAVEL OR GO ON A VACATION?

Q: What if I have to travel or go on a vacation during the diet?

The tail-end of a vacation or holiday like Thanksgiving or Christmas is a great time to start the preload or Phase 1, the gorging phase! Enjoy eating as much as you like.

A tough time to begin Phase 2, the low-calorie phase, is over the holidays: do you really want to deny yourself a glass of champagne or a holiday meal with family and friends? You may have an abundance of enthusiasm to start your weight-loss journey, but don't let enthusiasm cloud your judgment.

Pick a date that will support, not hinder, your efforts. Can you find a block of time for your round that falls between holidays and vacations? Don't forget, you will also want to avoid sugars and starches for three weeks in Phase 4…

Holidays are hard, but traveling isn't so bad, right?

It's not easy to stick with the diet when you're traveling but it's still possible. I recommend prepping your food in plastic containers. I was traveling for a 1-week period and didn't have access to a kitchen. I would visit the grocery store and buy a bag of shredded cabbage, some grilled chicken breasts, or lean deli meat, and 0 calorie dressing and make a salad on the road. You can also buy boiled or pickled eggs and eat them without the yolk, snack on turkey jerky, canned tuna in water, plain Greek yogurt, and even protein bars and protein shakes (provided they have no sugar and are low in fat and net carbs). If you must eat out in a restaurant, just ask for a salad with a lean protein and request no dressing, no cheese, no avocado, and no nuts ("no fun"). You want to stay away from fats. Have a look at the list of Rogue Foods at the end of this book. You'll see there are quite a few options if you're willing to go off the original Simeons Protocol. I ate everything in the list of Rogue Foods and still lost weight.

If you need a 2-week or longer break from the diet due to holidays, illness, or some other reason, I recommend coming off the HCG hormone and going into Phase 4 Maintenance until you can resume the diet and medication. It is believed that staying on the medication while eating normally can cause a lot more weight gain.

HOW LONG DO I HAVE TO WAIT BEFORE DOING ANOTHER ROUND?

Q: How long do I have to wait before doing another Round?

It is normally recommended that you take longer and longer breaks between successive diet rounds. In the original Simeons Protocol, breaks are recommended as follows. Keep in mind, Dr. Simeons did not recommend patients lose more than 34 pounds in a round:

> *Patients requiring the loss of more than 34 lbs. must have a second or even more courses. A second course can be started after an interval of not less than six weeks, though the pause can be more than six weeks. When a third, fourth or even fifth course is necessary, the interval between courses should be made progressively longer. Between a second and third course eight weeks should elapse, between a third and fourth course twelve weeks, between a fourth and fifth course twenty weeks and between a fifth and sixth course six months. In this way it is possible to bring about a weight reduction of 100 lbs. and more if required without the least hardship to the patient.*

> \- Dr. Simeons, *Pounds and Inches*

Some people are quite successful with breaks as short as two weeks. However, I am of the opinion that it is a good idea to take *at least* one week off for every two weeks of dieting. At the minimum, I recommend going through the entire three weeks of Phase 4 plus three weeks of Phase 5 ("real life") before resuming another long round.

Breaks aren't only about flushing the hormone from your body: they have many physical and psychological benefits. Breaks also give you an opportunity to practice the skills of maintaining your weight, which is often harder than the diet itself.

Also note, that the faster you eat at your TDEE (Total Daily Energy Expenditure), the faster you will recover from the strains of dieting. If you continue to chronically undereat and lose weight once the round ends, you are still in a dieting state, and not recovering.

TDEE: Total Daily Energy Expenditure. The more active you are, the more calories you require to meet your daily energy needs. Your TDEE is your BMR + the calories you burn through activity. For example, if my BMR (Basal Metabolic Rate) is 1400 calories and I burn 100 calories walking and another 300 lifting weights, I will need to consume 1800 calories a day just to maintain my bodyweight.

*The tricky part to calculating your TDEE is being accurate with your activity level, neither over or underestimating. Most people overestimate their calories burnt through exercise. In fact, **a classic study of overweight individuals who self-perceived as 'diet resistant', found they had overestimated their energy expenditure by as much as 250***

*calories a day, and underreported
food intake by 1052 calories a day. ***

---

*Source:
http://www.nejm.org/doi/full/10.1056/NEJM199212313272701

Breaks between rounds are a great opportunity to develop a better relationship with food and practice maintaining a healthier body weight. Unfortunately, the temptation to overeat during a break is huge when you know you will be doing another round and you can easily drop any weight you gain. However, this kind of thinking ultimately takes you further away from your long-term weight-loss goal and can set you up for disordered eating cycles of indulging and restricting. When eating habits aren't changed and nothing is learned from the experience, the HCG Diet becomes a crutch.

Obesity experts suggest an initial weight loss goal of 10% of your starting body weight (to be lost over a six-month period) followed by a period of maintenance of not less than six months before trying to lose more. They believe this is the best way to prevent weight regain.

HOW DO I HANDLE SOCIAL VISITS?

Q: How do I handle social visits?

Social visits are tough! During one round, I spent five days at my aunt's house. She is the best cook I've ever known, and I was worried about 1) being rude by refusing her cooking 2) eating what she cooked and going off my diet 3) eating food I brought while everyone else ate a different meal and upsetting them.

After thinking carefully about the options, I decided to let her know in advance that I was on a diet, and what I could and couldn't eat. I didn't want to be a burden to her, so I brought food with me and kept it in the fridge: deli meat, apples, and a spinach-egg frittata I'd made in advance.

I was more worried than I had to be.

My aunt was very supportive, and even poached some salmon in her sous-vide, to keep it tender and juicy without adding any sauces and extra calories. She served it with steamed vegetables and we all ate the same thing (though I skipped the potatoes). She gave me a jar of home-made pickles and offered me fresh garden vegetables and fruit.

I also had friends and family to visit over those five days, and I let them all know I was on a diet. It really took the pressure off of saying no to snacks and meals during visits. They respected my choices and didn't force food on me. I highly recommend sharing your goals with your family and friends. When you phrase it as a specific goal "I'm trying to lose 20 pounds" rather than a diet, "I'm on the HCG Diet" it's something concrete and relatable.

When I told my friends and family about what I could and couldn't eat on the diet, I didn't mention I was on the HCG Diet. I simply told them I was eating vegetables, fruits, and lean proteins each day, and not eating any butter, oil, sugars, or starches. It was just simpler that way.

HOW DO I DEAL WITH CRITICS?

Q: How do I deal with critics?

After I lost twenty pounds, a few people told me I looked great and didn't need to diet. I was flattered but also surprised: I was still officially overweight and only half-way to my goal. Could they not see that I was carrying an extra twenty pounds on my 5'6" frame?

Guess what? The same people that told me I didn't have to lose anymore weight were also obese.

Sometimes, making healthy changes to our lives can feel threatening to friends and family members because it forces them to examine their own unhealthy habits. Also, if our goals conflict with other people's lifestyle choices, there can be tension. Don't be surprised if not everyone supports you in your weight-loss goals.

I am fortunate that my husband was always 100%

supportive of my goals and loved me no matter what I weighed. But I also know how hard it can be to stay on track when your efforts are criticized or minimized by others.

My advice is to keep your eye on the prize and surround yourself with people who will support you in your weight-loss journey, whether that's on Facebook or in an HCG Diet forum, or someone you can call up now and again for support such as a coach or friend. If you can find someone to do the diet with, even better!

Stay positive and if your friends have any fears about this diet, tell them to read this book.

* * *

Let me tell you a story; it's not uncommon. A friend of mine tried the HCG Diet (kind of, sort of, not really.) She did the injections but quit after one week. She said she was "starving", even though she was eating more calories than the original plan called for. However, she didn't do a preload, and she didn't follow the food plan. Nor did she attempt to adjust her dosage up or down. To be fair, she didn't even know that she could adjust her dosage. She told me, "I didn't do the preload. Didn't follow the instructions. I was starving and felt super wired and it gave me bad insomnia. I hated it, but some people swear by it." Sadly, this was her first and probably her last experience on the HCG Diet, and she's still bitter about it. This is very common amongst people who have tried the diet and given up, not because the diet failed them but because they failed to follow the diet. Her verdict, "I decided it wasn't healthy."

Unfortunately, she didn't really do the diet, but now has some very strong opinions about it. You will encounter this a lot online: lots of critics and experts with strong opinions, but no real personal experience on the HCG Diet OR people who have done the HCG Diet (and quite possibly other diets and diet pills) too many times and claim it wrecked their metabolism.

All I can say is, ignore the naysayers and give this diet a try for three weeks. If you've struggled to lose weight in the past, this may be your last diet, ever.

Pick a protocol and commit 100%. Do Phases 1, 2, 3, and 4 properly. You will be amazed by the results.

You can do this.

WILL I BE HUNGRY?

Q: Will I be hungry on the HCG Diet?

I'm going to keep it real. Not everyone feels hungry, but I certainly had my moments.

> *If you've had a history of undereating or an eating disorder, it is possible that your hunger signals are off, and you don't get the same hunger signals that other people do.*

Chances are, you will feel hunger at various times on the

diet, and often towards the end of a round. In those situations, I found drinking water or having a cup of coffee or green tea helped immensely. Extra protein was also very helpful, especially on days I was more physically active. Sometimes, I would simply distract myself until the hunger would pass.

Regardless, the HCG hormone should prevent hunger, as long as the dosage is correct. You may wish to adjust your dosage down every time you lose 15 – 20 pounds. Too little or too much hormone can cause extreme hunger and I have experienced both!

Your hunger should be mild, and manageable. If not, talk to your doctor and consider adjusting your dosage.

The first week of the HCG Diet is often the hardest for people. Your body is adjusting to fewer carbs and calories and dumping its glycogen stores. Stick with it: the discomfort will pass, and you will feel good again.

CRAVINGS AND EMOTIONAL EATING

Q: Will I still have cravings?

If you're on the right amount of HCG, you may feel mild hunger at times, but you should never feel like you're starving. Hence, the HCG Diet can be a valuable tool for making you aware of the difference between real hunger and emotional hunger, aka cravings.

For example, I wouldn't feel "hungry" until I would go grocery shopping and walk through the baked goods section. Seeing all those delicious pastries could trigger my cravings. It wasn't real hunger though, because the desire would vanish once I left the store. I recommend the book, *Weight Loss Apocalypse: Emotional Eating Rehab Through the HCG Protocol* by Robin Phipps Woodall for more information on this topic. I especially recommend using her hunger scale in Phase 4 as a way to manage the problem of overeating.

> *You can also search "hunger scale" online; there are lots of versions available. However, I don't recommend using a hunger scale in Phase 2 of the diet as the hormone may prevent you from feeling hungry enough to eat!*

Being on the HCG Diet really helped put me in touch with my hunger cues as well as my cravings and triggers. It was a chance to experience true hunger and distinguish it from mouth hunger, which is simply wanting a taste of something even though your stomach is full.

Some people find they have less cravings on a low-carb or ketogenic diet. There are HCG Diet versions such as Dr. Zach LaBoube's HCG 2.0 that advocate a ketogenic approach. Many people have been successful with an ultra-low carb diet, though I think it is best suited for sedentary individuals.

A low-carbohydrate diet is defined as an eating plan consisting of less than 20% of a day's calories from carbohydrate, or 20 – 60 grams a day. Although low-carb diets are currently popular, a randomized, controlled trial published in the New England Journal found that while a low-carbohydrate diet provided a significantly greater weight loss in six months (7%) than a traditional, high-carbohydrate calorie restricted diet (3%), no difference between groups could be detected after 12 months. In fact, the most successful diet for keeping the weight off appears to be a high-protein diet, where 30% of the calories come from protein. Individuals report feeling fuller and experience less hunger while consuming fewer calories.

Personally speaking, a low-carb diet has a negative impact on my athletic performance, mood, mental acuity, and energy. I didn't feel good on less than 70 grams of carbs a day while dieting and taking HCG. I also think removing fruit from your diet means you will miss out on important nutrients and vitamins you can't get easily from other foods. However, some people love a ketogenic diet (less than 50 grams of carbs) and feel good on it. Since every body is different, you may wish to experiment with this.

Hunger tips

Q: Do you have some tips for dealing with hunger?

I recommend keeping a journal throughout your HCG Journey to note any foods that 1) satisfy your hunger, and 2) trigger it.

For me, a cup of coffee or green tea, or chugging a liter of water could really get me over a hungry moment or buy me a half-hour until meal-time. Sometimes, if I'd eaten all my food for the day and was still hungry, a bit of plain fat-free Greek yogurt would help. I encourage you to reflect a little on what works for you.

Also, I encourage you to eat more protein. If you're doing the original Simeons Protocol, you can double your protein portions and still lose weight. Protein is the most satiating (filling) of all the macronutrients. One of my favorite snacks was a 5-calorie pickle wrapped in lean deli meat with mustard and lettuce.

Don't forget to drink at least half your bodyweight in ounces of water each day because thirst often masquerades as hunger.

If hunger persists for more than a couple of days, ask yourself:

1. Did I do a proper preload in Phase 1 and eat to capacity every day for 2 - 3 days before starting the low-calorie phase?
2. Do I have the right dosage?
3. Am I using real prescription HCG hormone?

4. Am I eating foods that trigger more hunger or cravings?
5. Am I exercising too much?
6. Am I getting enough sleep?
7. Are my emotional needs taken care of?
8. Am I eating too little and do I need to add more protein?
9. Is this the right time for me to be dieting?
10. Have I been dieting for too long, and is "diet fatigue" setting in?

Stomach Growls

The fact that your stomach is growling is no indication of hunger. Doctors call this "borborygmi" (pronounced *BOR-boh-RIG-me*), and the truth is, it doesn't come from your stomach at all. It is simply excessive gas moving in your intestines. Be sure to chew your food more slowly to reduce the amount of air in your intestines.

HOW DO I PREVENT A WEIGHT LOSS STALL?

Q: How do I prevent a weight-loss stall?

A weight-loss stall is the point at which you are not losing any more weight. A stall can last several days, and it can be a demoralizing experience. (Note: not losing weight for a day is not really a weight loss stall.)

Rest assured, it is entirely normal to experience a weight-loss stall because people don't lose weight in a linear fashion. We can drop two pounds overnight, then nothing, then lose a half pound, then we may even gain a little, then whoosh! we suddenly drop a pound or two. Different things are going on in the body as it burns up fat reserves and removes waste material, and it's important to stay the course and not get upset: the weight will come off.

Why Stalls Happen

A weight-loss stall often occurs at various times throughout the diet: most people experience a stall only five days into the diet, once they've lost several pounds. Individuals may also plateau or stall after the first 15 pounds have been lost. Almost everyone experiences a stall towards the end of a round: the body simply needs to "catch up".

Weight-loss stalls can be the result of 1) too few calories so the body goes into "starvation mode", 2) not enough activity, 3) hitting a previous set-point, 4) the body recalibrating to its new weight and "catching up", 5) constipation, 6) water retention, 7) hormonal fluctuations, and 8) inflammation due to unusual amounts of exercise. Consider these reasons and address any issues as needed.

CAN I EXERCISE ON THE DIET?

Q: Can I exercise while I'm on the diet?

Absolutely! Walking is a great activity, since the pumping action of your legs helps to move lymphatic fluid and waste material around. This can help you lose more weight and flush out toxins.

If you're already active, keep doing what you're doing. You may have to dial down the volume or intensity a bit though or increase your calories slightly on your more active days.

Keep in mind that increasing your activity beyond normal levels will likely result in more hunger.

I'M CONSTIPATED. WHAT CAN I DO?

Q: I'm constipated. What can I do?

Because you're eating so much less, and the diet lacks fiber and fats, you may find yourself only having a bowel movement every two to three days. If you haven't had a movement in three days, you have a few options:

- Increase the amount of water you're drinking.
- Add in some electrolytes (ones that don't contain sugar).
- Increase fiber by eating more vegetables.
- Increase your exercise and activity levels.
- Eliminate aspartame, sugar alcohols, and artificial sweeteners, which may cause constipation in some people.
- Double up on Magnesium

If those don't work, you could try a tea called "Smooth Move" for some gentle overnight relief. You can also try MiraLAX. In severe cases, you may wish to use a suppository or something like Exlax. If you are still having problems, talk to your doctor. I realize that the original protocol only recommends suppositories, but I have had positive results with the tea, MiraLAX and Exlax even if they are "off protocol". (I especially recommend the tea, since it has zero calories, or MiraLAX, since it is gentler.)

Just don't depend on supplements too much; overreliance on laxatives can shut down your ability to have a natural bowel movement.

CAN I USE MAKEUP AND LOTION?

Q: Can I use makeup and lotion?

The original Simeons' Protocol doesn't permit the use of cosmetics, lotions, and creams but most modern protocols permit them. It is possible that the reason they weren't permitted 70 years ago is that it was very common for these products to contain animal fats such as lard or tallow. Nowadays, it is more common for products to use plant-based ingredients. Regardless, I continued to use face creams, cosmetics, and body lotions throughout my rounds.

From the book, *Pounds and Inches*, Simeons writes:

> *We are particularly averse to those modern cosmetics which contain hormones, as any interference with endocrine regulations during treatment must be absolutely avoided. Many women whose skin has in the course of years become adjusted to the use of fat containing cosmetics find that their skin gets dry as soon as they stop using them. In such cases we*

permit the use of plain mineral oil, which has no nutritional value. On the other hand, mineral oil should not be used in preparing the food, first because of its undesirable laxative quality, and second because it absorbs some fat-soluble vitamins, which are then lost in the stool. We do permit the use of lipstick, powder and such lotions as are entirely free of fatty substances. We also allow brilliantine to be used on the hair but it must not be rubbed into the scalp. Obviously sun-tan oil is prohibited.

— Dr. Simeons, *Pounds and Inches*

CAN I CHEAT ON THE DIET?

Q: Can I cheat on the diet?

Of course you can. Cheating or going off-plan happens to almost everyone at some point. However, there are better and worse ways to "cheat" and how well you cheat can determine whether you will experience a weight-loss stall or gain, and how pronounced it will be. .

If you are going to cheat and eat more calories, then choose lean proteins over carbs, and carbs over fats. Stick with a high-protein snack if possible. Do your best to avoid fats, sugars, and starches. Remember, the diet is usually three to six weeks long, a very short time to go without these things.

If you feel a cheat coming on, I recommend giving yourself 20 minutes: leave the room, go for a walk, have a shower, or distract yourself in some way. You may find the moment passing. If it doesn't, and you still want to cheat, ask yourself: "How will I feel about myself in an hour if I eat this, right now?" If you can live with yourself, go ahead.

A word about alcohol: I do not recommend drinking any alcohol on this diet. The reason is that alcohol is metabolized as both a fat and a carbohydrate in the body and is devoid of vitamins and nutrients (in fact, it even interferes with nutrient absorption!) You will be consuming so few calories on the diet that you need every micronutrient you can get from food. The other problem with drinking is that it can reduce your willpower and make it more likely for you to cheat on the diet.

The problem with cheating is that it can be very hard to stop once you start. If you do cheat, try to stay within your calories for the day. Whatever you do, don't punish yourself by eating a lot less food the next day, or doing extra exercise: that will just make things worse for you on this diet. Have your cheat and get back on track as soon as possible.

GOOD SOURCES OF PROTEIN

Q: What are some good sources of lean protein?

Lean proteins that are low in fat and relatively low in carbohydrates include, but are not limited to:

- 100 grams COOKED chicken breast = 31 grams of protein.
- 100 grams CANNED tuna in water = 24 grams of protein.
- 1 cup non-fat cottage cheese = 24 grams of protein.
- 1 cup fat-free Greek yogurt = 23 grams of protein.
- 100 grams COOKED shrimp = 21 grams of protein.
- 1 cup or 752 grams of Eggbeaters = 21 grams of protein.
- 1 Kirkland protein bar = 21 grams of protein.
- 1 cup of Carb Master non-fat milk = 11 grams of protein.

Keep in mind that weighed protein is very different from protein macros. It's easy to get confused but 100 grams of cooked chicken breast yields about 31 grams of protein.

Nuts are a source of protein but are too high in fat and low in protein to include in this list. For example, 30 grams of walnuts contains 20 grams of fat and a mere 5 grams of protein. This means a handful of walnuts is about 200 calories!

Beans, legumes, and grains are considered – for macronutrient purposes – carbohydrates that are high in fiber and low in protein.

WHEN SHOULD I COME OFF THE HCG DIET?

Q: When should I come off the diet?

You should come off the diet if:

1. You have reached your goal.
2. You don't want to get any leaner.
3. You need a break.
4. You find yourself binging or unable to stay on the diet.
5. You're not getting results, and you can't figure out why.
6. You can't function at work.
7. You've become a very difficult person to be around, and your work and relationships are suffering.

Take a break and do another round at a later time.

Of course, if you feel unwell at any time, or are experiencing strange symptoms, talk to your HCG Diet physician.

CHAPTER 3: LIST OF ROGUE FOODS

Here is a list of rogue foods that are considered "off-protocol" and not permitted in the original Simeons Diet. I enjoyed every one of them and still lost weight.

- 0-calorie salad dressings
- A tablespoon of milk, 3x a day in my coffee
- Brewers Yeast
- Carb Blocker Protein Milk
- Chicken bratwurst
- Chicken sausage
- Cocoa powder
- Diet soda
- Fat-free cheese
- Frozen mixed berries
- Garlic aioli mustard
- I enjoyed zucchini, kale, mushrooms, green beans, broccoli, snow peas, bamboo shoots, red and yellow peppers, artichokes, asparagus and any basically any vegetable that wasn't starchy (although I had sweet potato and white potatoes a couple times)
- Jimmy Dean turkey sausage
- Lake-caught fish
- Light cream cheese

- Lime juice
- Miracle noodles
- Mixing more than two vegetables in a meal to create a salad, stir-fry, or frittata (I always did this)
- Pickles
- Protein bars*
- Protein powder*
- Protein shakes
- Reddi Egg
- Sauerkraut
- Splenda
- Sprouted bread on occasion
- Sriracha
- Soy sauce
- Sugar-free coffee creamer such as Salted Caramel, Peppermint, or Hazelnut
- Sugar-free Jell-O
- Sugar-free pudding mix
- Unsweetened almond milk
- Vegetable spray for cooking

*I found Quest and the Kirkland brand of protein bars at Costco to be best suited to the diet as they each have 20 grams of protein and are low fat and don't contain any sugar. Each bar has about 22 grams of carbs, but this includes 14 grams of fiber, which means the body only absorbs about 8 carbs (also referred to net carbs). As for protein powder, I enjoyed a whey isolate-casein mix called Combat Powder from Costco. It is Cookies and Cream flavoured, and low in fat and carbs.

CHAPTER 4: IMPORTANT TERMINOLOGY

Your knowledge of the HCG Diet and nutrition will vastly increase if you familiarize yourself with the following terms. Even if you are an experienced HCG Dieter, you may learn a few things! I've tried to present the information in a logical order.

HCG V1.0, The Original Simeons Protocol – Dr. Simeons pioneered the original HCG Diet in the 1950s after successfully treating thousands of obese patients at his in-patient clinic in Rome, Italy. Daily injections of HCG (125 IU) were given and dieters were restricted to less than 500 calories a day and ate from a small list of permitted foods. No fats were allowed during the diet phase. Activity was limited to light walking.

Thousands of people still follow the original protocol as outlined in his book, *Pounds and Inches*.

HCG v2.0 - Dr. Zach LaBoube is the author and creator of "HCG 2.0". HCG 2.0 advocates more of a ketogenic approach: more protein, less carbohydrates, but still no fats during the diet phase because the hormone (in theory) makes you very sensitive to fats. There is more flexibility regarding foods you can eat but carbs are limited to less than 30 grams a day. Calories are higher and calculated for each individual based on their BMR. Dr. Zach LaBoube sells the homeopathic drops on his website, which he believes are as good as prescription-grade HCG products you get from a pharmacy.

Phase 1 – The Pre-Diet or Loading Phase of any protocol. This is where you eat to capacity for two to three days while taking your medication. It is extremely important to eat as much as possible (without making yourself sick) during this time. This helps to rev up your metabolism for the next phase and helps to minimize cravings and hunger in the first week of Phase 2. The extra fats are also believed to help spread the HCG hormone throughout the body. It sounds counter-intuitive: "Eat to lose!" but it works.

> *Don't worry about gaining weight in Phase 1: most people lose all their loading weight in the first two to three days of Phase 2. Those that are diligent about eating as much as they can handle usually experience the most weight loss, and this is exactly what happened to me. After gorging myself for 3 days, I gained 5 pounds. Once I started Phase 2, I lost 6.8 pounds in 2 days.*

Phase 2 – The Very Low-Calorie Phase. In Phase 2, you normally consume 500 – 1000 calories a day in conjunction with your HCG medication. Phase 2 usually lasts 23 – 43 days, give or take a few days. The first two to five days are the hardest and often hungriest as your body adjusts to lower calories and the hormone has not yet reached its full effect. After that, you're not as hungry and your energy improves.

Phase 2/3 – I prefer to refer to this stage as Phase 3, as it represents a new phase of the diet. However, Phase 3 is traditionally referred to as simply the end of Phase 2. It only lasts three days. You stop taking the medication, so it can clear your system while you continue to follow the Phase 2 diet. According to Dr. Simeons, "This is a very essential part of the treatment, because if they (patients) start eating normally as long as there is even a trace of HCG in their body they put on weight alarmingly at the end of the treatment." Your weight on the last day of this stage becomes your new setpoint, a weight you want to maintain within two pounds (if you aren't trying to gain muscle).

Phase 3/4 – Traditionally referred to as Phase 3, this is a 3-week period where calories are increased. Dr. Simeons said individuals are free to eat anything they please except sugars and starches. He believed avoiding sugars and starches during this time is crucial to keeping the weight off and creating a new set point for your body. For Phase 3 (what I prefer to call Phase 4), he advocated keeping your weight within two pounds of your last day on Phase 2/3. If you do gain more than two pounds, he advised doing what is called an "Apple Day". (That is not my personal recommendation.)

Phase 4/5 or The rest of your life – The diet is over.

Your weight should be stable, and you can reintroduce sugars and starches. Start small, and don't binge or you'll gain the weight back. You now have a great opportunity to experiment with foods you used to eat and see how your body responds. You may find that certain foods you used to eat cause you to gain weigh immediately, or that you feel poorly when you eat or drink certain items. Watch for food sensitivities: if you experience symptoms such as immediate bloating, gas, or diarrhea, you may want to avoid or restrict those items in the future. Your taste buds will have also changed; you may even find yourself craving new, healthier foods!

P1, P2, P3, P4 – Phase 1, Phase 2, Phase 3, etc.

VLCD – Very Low-Calorie Day. If you are following the original version of the HCG Diet, you will only consume 500 calories per day. Phase 2 is made up of 21 – 42 VLCD's, possibly more. You may hear people say VLCD1, VLCD2, referring to which day they are on.

LCD – Low Calorie Day. On some versions of the HCG Diet, you consume more than 500 calories per day, which is considered "Low Calorie".

R1, R2 – Round 1, Round 2, etc... Every time you do a "round" of the HCG Diet, you add another number to the R.

Putting it all together, if someone says they are on R1, P2, VLCD10 it means they are on Round 1, Phase 2, Very Low-Calorie Day

10 of the HCG Diet.

Apple Day – In the original version of the HCG Diet, if you gain more than two pounds during maintenance, you are instructed to immediately do an Apple Day. You eat six large apples over a 24-hour period, beginning at lunch and continuing until lunch the next day. You are only allowed to drink water (no other fluids). Dr. Simeons said this should put you back in your desired weight range.

Steak Day – A steak day is another option to put you back in your desired weight range if you gain more than two pounds during maintenance. To do a Steak Day, eat nothing all day and just drink plenty of water, coffee and/or tea. For dinner, you are instructed to eat a huge steak (8 - 14 oz.) plus an apple or raw tomato. Chicken breast meat can be substituted for steak.

Clean Load – Some protocols recommend minimizing your sugars and carbs and prioritizing fats, proteins, and low carb vegetables and even eliminating fruit during your preload (Phase 1). The theory is that this helps to reduce sugar and carb cravings during the diet phase and gets you into ketosis (fat burning mode) faster. Some people also prefer a clean load because they gain less weight in Phase 1 (1 – 4 pounds). This is mainly due to the fact that clean loaders consume fewer carbs and therefore accumulate much less water during their load.

Do carbs make you gain weight? Well, there's a reason for that. Every gram of carbohydrate

> *attracts roughly 3 grams of water, which will make you heavier – not necessarily fat. You'll notice that as soon as you drop your carbs in Phase 2, you'll shed a lot of water in the first few days. The more carbs you've eaten, the more water weight you can expect to "lose".*

Dirty Load – This is where you eat as much as you want of any food you like during the preload (Phase 1). A dirty load is fun for the first day or two but can feel gross if you overindulge. The theory is that eating as much as you want of anything you like will reduce future cravings and kill the desire for junk food later. Some people say a dirty load is more effective than a clean load when it comes to losing weight, but this may be due to all the water they've gained from eating so many carbs. It is not unusual to gain 5 – 10 pounds on a dirty load, only to have it melt off in the first few days of the diet. It's dramatic, and satisfying, to see the scale go down so fast but it is less about fat loss and more about shedding the extra water weight.

Ketogenic Diet – A true ketogenic diet consists of about 70 – 75% of its daily caloric intake from fat, 20% from protein and only 5% from carbohydrates. It is a high-fat, ultra-low carb diet.

Ketosis – When your body doesn't have enough carbohydrates from food sources, it burns fat instead. This process is called ketosis. Ketosis usually kicks in after three to four days of eating less than 50 grams of carbohydrates a day. Some people have to eat even fewer carbohydrates (less than 30 grams) and can take up to 2-3 weeks to get into ketosis.

Keto-flu – Many people complain of brain fog, l
and cold or flu-like symptoms while their body adapts to a
ketogenic or low-carb diet. Symptoms can last from three
days to several weeks.

Any diet that puts you in a caloric-deficit will cause you to burn fat, but ketosis is a metabolic process where the body depletes its glycogen storage and is forced to adapt to fat as a primary source of fuel in the absence of carbs.

Keto Strips – There are three main ketone bodies that are excreted from the body during ketosis. Acetoacetate is one of the ketones that is produced early in a ketogenic diet and can be easily measured by dipping the ketone paper test strips into your urine. The results on the test strip are color coded, with darker colors indicating higher amounts of ketones. Because the keto strips only test for one ketone, you may be in ketosis even if the strips don't indicate it.

Low Carb – A low-carb diet is when you drop carbs below 150 grams per day. Ultra-low carbs are when you drop your carbs below 50 grams a day. Most ketogenic diets are considered ultra-low carb. (Most North Americans average between 225-325 grams of carbs per day on a 2000-calorie diet.) Note that fruits, vegetables, sugars, and starches are all forms of carbohydrates.

Net Carbs – If you look at an ingredients label, you will see grams of Total Carbohydrates. In order to calculate the Net Carbs of a product, simply subtract the grams of fiber from the total carbohydrates listed on the label. For example, if a protein bar has 22 grams of Total Carbs and 15 are from Fiber, the Net Carbs are 7.

Fiber - Fiber is a carbohydrate that the body can't easily digest. It helps promote regular bowel movements and a healthy gut biome. Because the amount of food you eat on the HCG Diet is so low, you will likely be consuming below the recommended daily intake of fiber each day, which is 25 – 30 grams a day.

Glycemic Load – Measures the impact that different carbohydrates have on the body and blood sugar. Food with a low glycemic load can make it easier to lose weight, prevent insulin resistance, and lower the risk of heart disease. Note that you can reduce the glycemic impact of a snack or meal by combining high glycemic items (such as dessert) with other foods are high in protein, fiber, and water.

The 10:1 Rule: This is not something I've ever come across in the HCG Diet, but I think it's helpful for managing your nutritional choices in Phase 2 and beyond. Research from the Harvard School of Public Health recommends a simple trick when it comes to choosing a product: the 10:1 Carbs to Fiber ratio. Essentially, for every 10 grams of carbohydrates in a product, there should be at least 1 gram of fiber. The lower the first number and the higher the second, the better: you have less chance of spiking your blood sugar and creating an insulin response.

For example, 10:2 is better than 10:1, and 5:2 is even better.

Eating a piece of fruit versus drinking fruit juice is much better for your blood sugar. The glycemic load is much lower because the fiber slows down the rate of sugar absorption in your bloodstream. To maintain your new weight after the diet is over, try to eat more unprocessed foods such as whole grains, vegetables, and fruit.

And on the subject of fruit juice, did you know that a serving of cranberry juice will spike your blood sugar faster than a Coca Cola? Google Glycemic Index and learn what foods and beverages might be sabotaging your weight loss.

BMR – Basal Metabolic Rate. Also referred to as RMR or Resting Metabolic Rate.

BMR is the number of calories a person burns in a day, at rest. BMR is responsible for approximately 60 to 70% of the total number of calories you burn in a day, not including physical activity. Having a high BMR means you get to eat like a teenager and not gain weight. Your BMR depends on a variety of factors like your age, height, gender, hormone health, and muscularity. For example, a 25-year-old man might burn more than 1800 calories a day (at rest) while a 40-year-old woman might burn 1400 calories a day (at rest).

Your BMR (aka metabolism) drops as you age and if you diet for extended periods of time. If you lose muscle, either due to lack of activity, bedrest, or severe calorie restriction, your BMR will also drop.

Diet Break: A diet break is also referred to as a "deload" in bodybuilding circles. In bodybuilding circles, it's typically done after a *minimum* of four weeks of intense dieting and provides several physical and psychological benefits. Diet breaks are also recommended for the HCG Diet.

Dr. Simeons believed a diet break would prevent an immunity to the hormone. He believed that after 40 injections, an immunity would build up and it would take about six weeks before the immunity would be lost, and the HCG would become fully effective again. If patients had a lot of weight to lose, they should do a six-week round, take a break, and then do another round, which he refers to as a "course" in his book.

From Dr. Simeons' book, *Pounds and Inches*, "When a third, fourth or even fifth course is necessary, the interval between courses should be made progressively longer. Between a second and third course eight weeks should elapse, between a third and fourth course twelve weeks, between a fourth and fifth course twenty weeks and between a fifth and sixth course six months. In this way it is possible to bring about a weight reduction of 100 lbs. and more if required without the least hardship to the patient."

Diet breaks on HCG are often taken during holidays, vacations or between rounds of HCG. During a diet break, HCG is stopped, and enough calories are eaten to maintain your bodyweight. A diet break is recommended when you are unable to stay on the protocol, regardless of the reason.

Dieting and restriction is hard, and takes it toll, physically and psychologically. You may get better results from doing several short rounds of HCG, with shorter diet breaks between rounds. Some people, like myself, have taken breaks as short as two weeks before resuming another round.

Binging – Binging is eating uncontrollably over a short period of time even in the absence of hunger. Binges can be planned or unplanned and are accompanied by feelings of guilt and shame. If you find yourself binging and unable to stay on the HCG Diet despite promises to yourself to get back on track day after day, then it is best to terminate your round early. Binging is a psychological disorder and should be addressed with a specialist. Binge eating can also be brought on by rigid dieting which is why the HCG Diet is not recommended for anyone with a history of disordered eating (unless carefully supervised).

Cravings - Giving into a craving doesn't constitute a binge episode, provided you limit yourself to that item and get back on track right away. Cravings can occur for a variety of legitimate reasons including emotional triggers, lowered leptin, hormonal imbalances, a bad batch of HCG, insufficient amounts of HCG, lack of sleep, or dieting for too long. If you are struggling with cravings or hunger on the HCG Diet, you may wish to 1) consider your emotional triggers and find ways to eliminate them or at least deal with them better, 2) get more sleep 3) change your dosage, 4) change your medication, 5) address hormonal issues with your doctor, 6) dig deep for motivation, 7) find a coach or support buddy, 8) take a diet break.

> *Stress impacts hormones, like cortisol, which can boost your appetite and lead to cravings. Since dieting is stressful, it can increase cortisol, which is why shorter rounds of HCG may be better if you find yourself struggling to stay on protocol. Not everyone is a good candidate for the HCG Diet or suited for a long round.*

Macros: Macronutrients make up the caloric value of food and getting enough (and not too much) of certain macros is essential to your health and body composition goals.

Essentially, all food is made up of three building blocks: carbohydrates, protein, and fats. These are what is referred to as macros. Some coaches consider alcohol to be a fourth macro, because of the way it is metabolized in the body (like a carbohydrate and a fat).

In order of importance on the HCG Diet:

Protein – the amino acids in protein helps build muscle and prevent muscle loss while dieting. Protein also helps control appetite and staves off hunger. Meat, fish, egg whites, dairy products and protein powders are excellent sources of protein. Every gram of protein has 4 calories.

Carbohydrates – the body and brain's preferred source of energy. They are stored in the liver, muscles as glycogen. Sources include fruit, vegetables, grains, sugar, and many processed foods. Some carbs are healthier than others, especially ones that are unprocessed and contain more fiber and nutrients. Every gram of carbohydrates has 4 calories.

Fats – are essential to hormone function, brain health, vitamin absorption, and healthy skin. Fats can come from oils, nuts, nut butters, fatty meats, and dairy products. Every gram of fat has 9 calories.

Some fats are healthier than others and trans-fats (the kinds of fats found in many processed foods to increase shelf life) should be avoided entirely. Saturated fats (the kinds of fats found in milk, butter, cheese, non-dairy creamer, coconut oil, and animal fats like lard) are an important of a balanced diet. According to the American Heart Association, saturated fats should not comprise more than 6% of your daily calories.

Alcohol – has 7 calories per gram.

Micronutrients: Vitamins and minerals like Vitamin A, potassium, and sodium are considered micronutrients. Different foods have different micronutrients. Micronutrients don't contain calories.

BMI – Stands for Body Mass Index. It is an outdated measurement that divides a person's mass by their height to give an inaccurate estimate of body fat based on population samples. It doesn't tell you anything about your specific body composition, such as how much muscle versus fat you may be carrying. This is why bodybuilders will always register as obese when BMI is used; it's a crude measurement that only factors in a person's weight.

DXA Scan -- The most accurate method for determining total body composition (muscle, bone, and body fat percentage) is a DXA scan. DXA stands for Dual Energy X-ray Absorptiometry. Other popular methods such as skinfold testing and bio-impedance devices are much less accurate at determining a person's bodyfat.

Intermittent Fasting - Intermittent Fasting gives people a smaller window to eat in a day, usually 8 - 10 hours, which can result in an overall decrease in calories. As an example, many people leave 14 hours between dinner and breakfast, having their last meal or snack at 8 pm and their first meal at 10 am. Though there is some debate, IF is reportedly good for inflammation, cellular repair, human growth hormone and insulin. Some people utilize Intermittent Fasting during their HCG Diet and beyond.

Maintenance: Maintenance is when you eat just enough calories to maintain your bodyweight.

Set-point: The weight at which your body likes to be at and can comfortably stay at with little effort. Phases 3 and 4, when done properly, help create a new set point for your body.

Reverse Dieting: This isn't a term used by the HCG Diet community, but it's practiced by bodybuilders after contest prep. Essentially, once you've ended a diet, you enter a "maintenance" phase where your body is getting used to its new weight set point. At this point, you can cautiously add in more calories, say 100 - 200 per week, and keep adding in more calories and tweaking the macros each week until you find yourself gaining weight. At that point, you back off and maintain your weight at the new caloric level. When done right, people who have only been able to consume 1400 calories in the past can find themselves able to eat a lot more calories (and carbs!) without gaining weight when they successfully reverse diet. Reverse dieting can be harder than the diet itself because it requires great discipline and strategy. Due to the possibility of unwanted weight gain, it is best to work with a nutritionist or coach like myself who specializes in reverse-dieting.

Whew! That's a lot of lingo for a diet. However, I did throw in some bonus nutritional information that I hope will serve you in P1, P2, P3 and beyond!

CONCLUSION: A BINGE ON FICTION, A STARVATION OF FACTS

What is the difference between fact and fiction? It's a good question in this era of fake news and dubious diet advice.

Simply put, fact is based not on opinion, but on events that are verified to be true, or, *have actually occurred,* regardless of the source.

The word fact comes from the Latin word "factum" meaning "something done".

While facts are considered verifiable, fiction is considered a product of the imagination.

As an example of things that sound medically plausible (especially given the source), but have no basis in fact, we have the Myth of the Falling Uterus.

For over 100 years, women were held back from many sports due to something called "The Myth of the Falling Uterus". It was believed that a woman's uterus would fall out if she competed in running races, played basketball, or ski jumped. So how did this myth come to be accepted as fact?

It likely dates back to the 1800s. Donald Walker first wrote a book called *Physical Exercises for Ladies* in 1836. In his book, he asserted that women should engage in "restrained and non-violent" exercise to protect their "peculiar function of multiplying the species."

Then in 1898, a German doctor wrote in a medical journal that "violent movements of the body can cause a shift in the position and a loosening of the uterus as well as prolapse and bleeding, with resulting sterility, thus defeating a woman's true purpose in life, i.e., the bringing forth of strong children.".

It may sound like pure fiction now, but the sources were respected, and the idea sounded feasible, and in time, this myth turned into a medical rationale to ban women from Olympic running events. On the basis of no scientific evidence whatsoever, women were not allowed to race distances longer than 200 meters until the 1960 Rome Olympics. And yet, even though there was never a record of a single falling uterus*, this medical myth continued to perpetuate for another 50 years.

Note that this is different from a prolapsed uterus and the National Institutes of Health does not list exercise as a probable cause of this medical condition.

Sources: *https://www.outsideonline.com/1783996/myth-falling-uterus* and *http://www.nytimes.com/1996/06/23/magazine/how-the-women-won.html*

Just how long did this myth persist? In 2010, Gian-Franco Kasper, president of the International Ski Federation, commented on ESPN that a woman's uterus could burst during a ski jump landing. This echoed a comment he had made in 2005 on NPR that ski jumping is "not appropriate for ladies from a medical point of view." For over a century, what we had was fiction masquerading as medical fact.

The moral of the story? "Trust but verify." Also, consider the source. None of these "experts" had any personal experience being a woman. Women had to compete in sports for decades before the Myth of the Falling Uterus could be laid to rest.

The HCG Diet also suffers more from too much fiction and not enough facts:

- Lose 1 – 2 pounds a day!
- Lose fat evenly!
- Preserve muscle!
- Reset your metabolism!
- Improve thyroid function!
- Keep the weight off permanently!

Only some of this is "true". As I've discussed in Chapter 2:

People can lose 1 - 2 pounds a day, but some days they will lose nothing, and the average weight loss is about a half a pound a day for women and slightly less than a pound a day for men.

You will not lose fat evenly. Your genetics determine

where you will pull the most fat.

You will probably lose some muscle as well as fat on the diet, but you can take steps to reduce muscle loss, such as eating more protein and stimulating muscle through exercise.

Your metabolism won't "reset" until you've kept the weight off for a period of at least 6 months or more.

Your thyroid function may improve if you have hypothyroidism. For example, my labs improved, and I decreased my dosage. However, this may also be due to the fact that I am a smaller person now, and I need a smaller dose. Body fat can certainly affect the way medication is absorbed.

Will you keep the weight off permanently? Only if you make the necessary lifestyle changes to eat smarter than you did before, whether that's reducing portion sizes or eating healthier.

The primary driving forces behind obesity and leptin resistance are an over consumption of highly palatable, high-calorie foods and beverages. Even overweight individuals that eat healthy tend to underestimate how much they consume. As mentioned previously, a classic study of overweight individuals who self-perceived as 'diet resistant', found they had overestimated their energy expenditure by as much as 250 calories a day, and (unknowingly) underreported food intake by 1052 calories a day.

This is why tracking food and weighing yourself daily may

be very helpful when you are trying to maintain your new weight, especially for the first few months as your body adjusts to its new set point.

Tracking doesn't have to be forever: you can ease off as you adopt new eating habits and find ways to maintain your new weight with ease. Since the research indicates that people who have kept the weight off long-term are highly active, it would benefit you to find an activity you enjoy, whether that's lifting weights, doing yoga, or walking every day. Besides burning calories, there are numerous mental and physical health benefits to exercise.

As you can see, the diet doesn't end with Phase 2. Keeping the weight off requires ongoing vigilance and behavior change, which gets easier with practice. For some, the joy of losing weight provides the motivation to keep going. For others, it can take multiple diet rounds to learn the lessons of permanent weight loss.

I have tried, in this book, to stick to the facts through real life experience and scientific evidence as far as the HCG Diet is concerned. This may come as a disappointment to some who are looking for a magic cure-all for obesity, but I have always preferred truth over deception. In the words of Gloria Steinem, "The Truth will set you free, but first it will piss you off." I imagine this book will garner some criticism, especially from those that make a living selling HCG products and services and exaggerating its benefits.

The HCG Diet is controversial, and over-hyped. Some of the information surrounding it has been scientifically tested while other information is simply conjecture and opinion. A person can go online, and cherry pick a study to support their personal viewpoint, but *science is based on the sum of the evidence* provided by the studies available. Anyone, including myself, should be willing to change his/her conclusions in light of new evidence. After all, science is about facts, not opinions.

My hope is that this book will spark a conversation and more research into the HCG Diet and how the hormone may help people to not only lose weight, but to do so more comfortably and successfully than other approaches.

Based on my personal experience with human chorionic gonadotropin, I believe there *is* something special about the hormone, but we need more quality-controlled studies to fully understand it.

Thank you for reading this book.

DID YOU ENJOY THIS BOOK?

I want to thank you for purchasing and reading this book. I really hope you got a lot out of it.

Can I ask a quick favor though?

If you enjoyed this book I would really appreciate it if you could leave me a positive review.

I love getting feedback from my customers and reviews on Amazon and Goodreads really do make a difference. I read all my reviews and would really appreciate your thoughts.

Thanks so much.

Adele Frizzell

ABOUT THE AUTHOR

Adele Frizzell is the author of several books. She has a Bachelor of Kinesiology and is an online health and fitness coach. At 45, she began to compete in powerlifting and won medals for her age and weight class. She believes that you can surprise yourself with what you can accomplish once you put your mind to it.

Adele loves to travel, hike, do yoga, lift heavy weights, and inspire people to get more out of life.

Please visit her website at www.AdeleFrizzell.com to learn more.

RECOMMENDED READING
In alphabetical order:

20 Essential Nutrition Habits for Permanent Weight Loss by Adele Frizzell

A 15-page guide on habits, mindset, and nutritional information to assist with health and weight maintenance. Download your free copy at www.AdeleFrizzell.com.

HCG Diet Options: Choosing Your Own Protocol by Lara Plagman

Lean Habits for Lifelong Weight Loss: Mastering Four Core Eating Behaviors to Stay Slim Forever by Georgie Fear, R.D.

Pounds and Inches: A New Approach to Obesity by A.T.W. Simeons, M.D.

Understanding Healthy Eating A Science-Based Guide to How Your Diet Affects Your Health by Renaissance Periodization

Weight-Loss Apocalypse: Emotional Eating Rehab Through the HCG Protocol by Robin Phipps Woodall

OTHER BOOKS BY ADELE FRIZZELL

The Cha Club Dating Man-ifesto

Are you tired of dating games? Having a hard time setting boundaries? Falling for the wrong kind of men? A fun, sisterly, kick-in-the-ass guide for women who feel unlucky in love. It includes 48 guidelines to help you weed out Mr. Wrong and find Mr. Right. I followed my own advice and found my husband less than a year later!

It's Not You, It's Us: A Guide for Living Together Without Growing Apart

Want more joy, intimacy, and respect in your relationship? Find out how to get the love you deserve in this inspiring and uplifting relationship guide for couples. A "relationship manual" you can return to time and again for a tune-up. Each chapter includes stories, homework, and activities to increase happiness and satisfaction. An indispensable book whether you're engaged, married, or living together!

Forty Daze: A Quest for Self-Improvement

What aspect of your life do you want to change? Small habits can lead to big changes as you'll see in this entertaining book on self-improvement and personal experiments. Learn some powerful tips and tricks to build new habits quickly and easily, including an "anchoring" technique developed by Dr. Fogg of Stanford University that has helped thousands of people to change their behavior.

Made in the USA
Lexington, KY
02 February 2019